CHAOS
to CURED

To a great man & friend.
I hope this helps to understand how much
your support has meant to me over the
past few years. I am always
there as a friend.

Warmly,
Kirk Miller

CHAOS
to CURED

The True Story of Defeating Bipolar Disorder

KIRK PATRICK MILLER

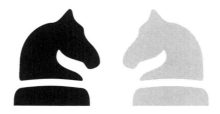

iUniverse, Inc.
Bloomington

CHAOS TO CURED
THE TRUE STORY OF DEFEATING BIPOLAR DISORDER

iUniverse books may be ordered through booksellers or by contacting:

iUniverse
1663 Liberty Drive
Bloomington, IN 47403
www.iuniverse.com
1-800-Authors (1-800-288-4677)

Because of the dynamic nature of the Internet, any web addresses or links contained in
this book may have changed since publication and may no longer be valid. The views
expressed in this work are solely those of the author and do not necessarily reflect the
views of the publisher, and the publisher hereby disclaims any responsibility for them.

Any people depicted in stock imagery provided by Thinkstock are models,
and such images are being used for illustrative purposes only.

Certain stock imagery © Thinkstock.

ISBN: 978-1-4759-7131-6 (sc)
ISBN: 978-1-4759-7132-3 (hc)
ISBN: 978-1-4759-7133-0 (e)

Library of Congress Control Number: 2013900528

Printed in the United States of America

iUniverse rev. date: 2/8/2013

PROFESSIONAL ENDORSEMENTS

➤ "After practicing medicine for over forty years, I never dreamed that one of my patients would discover the most effective method of treating bipolar. Since dealing with Kirk Miller, we still do not know if it is a complete cure or the treatment has kept his bipolar in a constant state of remission; however, the results I have seen with Mr. Miller and others who have undergone the same treatment are undeniable. I hope everyone will find Mr. Miller's memoir as inspiring and surprising as I found watching his recovery. I feel lucky to have been a part of a once-in-a-lifetime discovery."

—Dr. Robert Simon, MD

➤ "Kirk Miller's memoir provides important, if not vital, insight into the bipolar condition. After working with over two thousand different individuals throughout the world, all suffering from ADD, dyslexia, and bipolar syndrome, I can say, without reserve, that seldom, if ever, have I read such an in-depth and fascinating account of what it is like to be truly bipolar. The fact that the author has cured himself and discovered a potential cure has revolutionary implications. Kirk Miller needs to be heard and heard widely. I endorse his memoir with overwhelming enthusiasm."

—Jeffery Freed, MAT, author of *Right-Brained Children in a Left-Brained World*

➢ "We are parents of a son who has bipolar. He has been hospitalized five times. It broke our hearts as we would have to call the police and watch them beat him into submission and take him to the hospital. He would be in there for five to six weeks and would then come home heavily medicated and go into a depressive state for months. In 2010 we heard about Kirk. He has been such a blessing in our lives, extremely helpful and supportive to us and to our son. Our son is now two years with no bipolar symptoms. We will be forever grateful for Kirk. His book will give many bipolar sufferers hope and know that they are not alone and that they can have a 'normal' life. Thank you."

—Darrel and Dixie Navratil

➢ "Here is a book that I believe is one of a kind … The in-depth story that Mr. Miller shares is a rare look into the mind of a bipolar episode … I believe that Mr. Miller has indeed found a way out of the emotional and mental prison in which bipolar has incarcerated so many individuals. I would encourage anyone and everyone to read this memoir, especially if you know someone with bipolar."

—Debra Slackman, MA, clinical psychotherapist

➢ "Mr. Miller provides a unique insight into the inner workings of a bipolar person's heart and mind, from the perspective of someone who has experienced it before and after successful treatment. This book is a must-have resource for anyone who loves a bipolar person but has a hard time understanding how bipolar disorder affects his/her thinking, mood, and actions."

—Sheryl Gurrentz, coauthor of *If Your Child Is Bipolar: A Parent-to-Parent Guide to Living with and Loving a Bipolar Child*

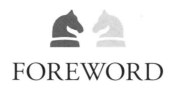

FOREWORD

Years ago I became a close friend to a young man who seemed "just" normal. I had known him since he was in elementary school and had stayed in contact as he grew into a man. He struggled from time to time with what I thought was depression, but it seemed "manageable." He fell in love with a wonderful young woman. They were married and had two great little boys. I was suddenly introduced to their reality when my friend was hospitalized in a catatonic state with a serious depression following an extreme manic period.

I visited him in the hospital and felt completely helpless; I can't imagine how his family felt. I learned that he had a long history of bipolar disorder that I had never suspected or even entertained as a possibility. Unfortunately, his family was not able to survive their bipolar ordeal, as they were never sure which person would be there on a given day.

Having been involved in the development of pharmaceuticals for most of my career, I looked into bipolar disorder to learn more about current treatment options, hoping to discover what I could do or advice I could offer to help my friend and his family. Almost all options seemed hopeless, and the treatments were very difficult for my friend, often providing no real help. I was confused and disturbed by how difficult this disorder is to identify and treat. I was further bothered by the lack of good pharmaceuticals for treatment.

Then I met Kirk Miller. He called me based upon a referral from a mutual friend. I was extremely skeptical, as my only point of reference was my friend and his constant battle with bipolar disorder. Kirk wanted my opinion of his personal experience with estrogen inhibitors and how they had helped him overcome his bipolar disorder. Kirk was interested in understanding what it would take to prove the benefit of using estrogen inhibitors in the treatment of bipolar sufferers and how he might best teach others about it. Over time, he earned my trust. I was impressed with his passion and persistence; he felt driven to give other sufferers their life back just as he had recovered his.

We spent time together talking about Kirk's experience and the results he and his doctor were seeing in other bipolar sufferers who were also trying estrogen inhibitors in their treatment. We also discussed ways to interest pharmaceutical companies and medical professionals in his experience and develop his treatment plan into a new and exciting option for doctors and future patients. In the end, we all agreed that telling Kirk's story to others was the best immediate option. I was impressed.

Most of us who have been impacted by or have observed bipolar disorder—also known as manic-depressive disorder—know that over the past decade many books and articles have been published dealing with bipolar disorder. Physicians, psychiatrists, and other health-care professionals have written important and detailed books defining and attempting to explain the condition. Others go into great detail describing historical and modern treatment strategies as well as ongoing research and clinical development. Current treatment strategies continue to be centered on drug cocktails, including mood stabilizers, such as lithium, dissociative anesthetics, and dopamine agonists. Many books and articles address more nontraditional approaches, including diet changes, dietary supplements, extreme diets, and stress reduction techniques.

Unfortunately, many individuals suffering from bipolar disorder, like my friend, find little success from any of these approaches or are dissatisfied by the significant side effects when they reach a stable condition. Many of these individuals are willing to take extreme measures to improve their condition, knowing that they have been told that bipolar disorder is managed but never cured.

Parents, family members, and friends of individuals suffering from bipolar disorder have also written books. They provide insights into the disease, including its destructive impact on families, relationships, and individuals suffering from the condition. Bipolar sufferers have also written about their paths, navigating both the ups and the downs as well as exploring treatments for their condition. Some victims offer stories of survival and struggles in managing the condition.

Some of these books are positioned as self-help books, written in an effort to help sufferers, family members, and friends cope with the condition and its destructive consequences. Although these books do offer comfort in just knowing that others have bipolar and are suffering, they do not really offer hope to the victims, their families, and their friends. Rather, the message all too often is about struggle and grief. What hope is seen is shallow or lacks a real, believable premise.

Chaos to Cured stands alone as a true, heartfelt telling of a dramatic realization that leads to a remarkable transformation sparked by determination and love. No one would ever want to live through the life experience described in this book; the details are just too hard. Yet the story and the ending create a true sense of hope for bipolar sufferers.

As Kirk relives his story, the reader not only is captivated but immediately understands that this book is a true story written with the passion and truth only a bipolar sufferer could convey. Kirk's story includes some aspect of all the other stories, treatments, and self-help strategies. It is clear that the grip the disease has on individuals with bipolar disorder, their family, and their friends cannot be underestimated, overlooked, or dismissed.

Chaos to Cured tells a chilling story of the struggles of a bipolar sufferer, his family, and his friends; but at the end there is an unexpected surprise. There is love, there is hope, and there is a future.

Dean P. Stull, PhD
Friend, Scientist, Entrepreneur and CEO

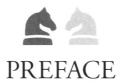

PREFACE

Against all odds and nearly dying in the process, I discovered a new method for treating and curing my bipolar disorder, a condition that had stifled my ability to connect to the world or to the people I cared most for and that had nearly cost me my life. My full recovery left my doctors, family, and friends in shock. A life that had been filled with chaos and pain was suddenly filled with love, calm, patience, success, and stability. In simple terms, my life became everything I had dreamed of, leading me to writing this memoir.

After watching friends, family, and acquaintances suffer with bipolar, losing their loved ones, friends, jobs, and even lives, I knew that keeping my discovery to myself would be selfish and wrong. Therefore, I am risking my professional reputation as a stable and honorable man to tell the world that there is hope for everyone currently struggling with this unique illness. I want nothing more than to help as many people as possible, and this memoir is the first step.

I am aware that my book will be highly controversial and many experts will challenge the truth of my claims. However, I am willing and ready for the world to examine every aspect of my life. The scrutiny will be worth it if it will inspire researchers to develop new standards of care for those with bipolar disorder and possibly other mental disorders.

Over the past five years, I have had the honor of working with amazing doctors and psychiatrists who have successfully used my method of treating the endocrine system with bipolar patients who had run out of all other options. We continued to see progress. I worked closely with the families and patients as a consultant and coach, as no one else could explain what they were going through. After growing close to many of these families and doctors, I was asked to write my life story and share it with the world. This memoir is not for me, although it was therapeutic to write. This memoir is dedicated to all the families and individuals who feel lost and hopeless. Research needs to be done, which is why I am donating all net profits from the sale of this book to Healing Unique Minds Foundation. My goal is to help people find the same happiness I now enjoy.

I hope everyone reading this memoir discovers a new understanding of what bipolar really is and how it affects the people whose lives it darkens, and I hope that the impossible hope for a cure is never out of reach, just sometimes hidden from view.

As a final note, I would ask everyone reading this memoir to keep in mind that I am no longer the man I once was, nor do I regret having bipolar. It may have adversely impacted my life in ways that I am unable to change, yet it was because of my illness that I risked my life to discover a new treatment that has forever changed my life and the lives of others for the better.

Although it took almost four years of data to convince anyone that there was something to what I had found, our continued success only makes me believe that this memoir is more important than my career or money. Life is not always predictable, but it is always filled with potential hope and happiness. My story may begin in darkness, but I would live the same life a thousand times over to discover the happiness and stability I now enjoy every day.

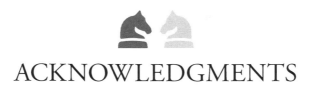

ACKNOWLEDGMENTS

:: Special Thanks ::

Words are unfit to convey the love and honor I feel for all those who have stood by me and forever changed my life for the better.

Dr. Robert Simon, I thank you for saving my life, as I would not be here without your skill, patience, and heart. To my mentor and friend who came to believe in me, Dean Stull, your contributions to the world, and to me, will never be forgotten.

I must also thank those involved with the formation of the Healing Unique Minds Foundation—Sheryl Gurrentz, Cindy Singer Abramson, Arif Gangji, and Richard Beck—as you have all given of yourselves while asking for nothing in return. I have never felt so honored to sit with such great minds and kind people.

To the amazing families and individuals I have had the pleasure to know and help, I believe that I can and will make a positive difference with the second chance I was given because of you. For that, I am forever in your debt.

To my family, which has always been loving and patient, I will continue to do my best to make you proud of the man I have become. I would not have survived without such strong people to guide and help me, especially my mother, who moved mountains in order to help me.

Dearest Nicoal, you will always be the light that led me to a new and fulfilling life. I have always believed in you, and I wish you the best in your life, wherever it may lead you.

Lastly, to anyone suffering with bipolar, this story is written for you and your families. I believe it will bring hope and warmth to all who read it.

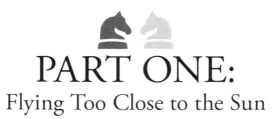

PART ONE:
Flying Too Close to the Sun

:: Mania's Flight and the Fall into Darkness ::

I.   MANIA AND SELF-MEDICATING

The moonlight sliced into the alleyway, its sharp lines making a beautiful contrast between everything it touched and the black shadows that I lay in. Opening my eyes, I stared up at the night sky. The stars were lost to the city lights, but the moon was full and bright, its cool blue hue making the alleyway seem cold. My head throbbed, and the world spun gently when I tried to move. The cold, hard cement I was lying upon felt oddly soothing, but even with all the alcohol and drugs flowing through my veins, my mind was still racing. I was twenty-one at the time, and even though I was still drunk and high, I was aching for drugs and alcohol. It would be a year until I was told that those feelings were related to what professionals called a manic episode. I was self-medicating in an attempt to slow the world down around me, but it wasn't working.

This was not the first time that a mixture of drugs and alcohol had left me passed out in a less-than-ideal location. I had woken up in worse and far more dangerous situations, yet I never thought anything about it. Not once did it occur to me that my actions were not those of a normal mind, especially when I was simply desperate to calm the unrelenting torrent of racing thoughts rushing through my mind. The world seemed bright, I felt powerful, and I had no ability to stay focused or any desire to rest.

Although I was now of legal drinking age, legality had never bothered me, and I had a history of using and selling drugs. To me, alcohol was a child's drug—not that I took any drug seriously, no matter what chemical or form of delivery. At the time, I had the potential to be a good person, but something had always steered me away from warmth and kindness. I was a selfish individual. Although I could be nice if it would benefit me, I could also be extremely cruel, having the ability to pick out someone's deepest insecurity and exploit it when I felt such insults were needed. I was lost to my own reality, and I didn't much care about myself, let alone anyone else.

Sitting up took more effort than I had expected, but slowly I lifted myself to my knees, leaning back and taking a deep breath of the cool night air. Looking back, this moment would have been perfect for self-examination, but at the time I didn't think twice. I thought I was doing great. My grades in college were good, I had quite a few romantic relationships that were flourishing, and I was working on a groundbreaking fiction manuscript that would bring me fame and fortune. I believed I was beyond brilliant and there wasn't anything on the planet that could keep me down.

With that thought, I smiled, my lips slightly crooked and my eyes wild as I stood up. Suddenly, I noticed that my right sleeve was torn and I had a deep scratch on my forearm that was deep enough to have left a trail of dried blood running down my forearm. I touched the deep scratch, running my fingers along the rough surface of the dried blood. A normal person might have paused to think about how he had ended up passed out in an alleyway, his shirt torn, and his right arm wounded. I, however, simply shrugged my shoulders and walked out of the shadows, ready to enjoy what was left of the waning night.

Walking out of the alleyway, I looked around, trying to find my bearings. The streets were empty except for a few homeless individuals wrapped in sheets and newspapers to protect them from the slight breeze that had picked up. I wasn't in the best section of Denver's downtown area. Although I remembered entering one of the more popular clubs with my friends, as well as drinking, I couldn't remember how or why I had wandered so far from the main strip of bars and clubs. Thinking back, it amazes me that I never questioned how I had ended up in an alleyway tucked in the shadows. At the time, however, I didn't pause to contemplate as I began walking toward the only main street I recognized. Though the night was quickly fading, I was still insistent on getting my fill of fun.

After walking for a few blocks, I heard my friend Mike's voice rise into the air. He was used to me doing wild things, but this time, his voice was laced with a hint of anger. "Kirk, I've been looking all over for you!" Turning around, I saw Mike running toward me. He was dressed in a stylish shirt, his hair spiked and highlighted. His long face was filled with a mixture of relief and frustration.

"What's wrong?"

Mike just stood there for a moment, staring at me as if I were crazy to ask. "Really? You have to ask?"

I could tell Mike was frustrated, but I turned back around and continued toward the street corner. Walking alongside me, Mike continued to talk, still surprised that I didn't remember anything. "Man, what the hell happened back there?"

"What are you talking about?" I asked as we crossed the empty street, a slight chill hitting my skin as the wind kicked up.

"You have to be kidding me," Mike said before laughing. I don't think he knew that I didn't remember; he probably thought I was just joking around. Feeling like I was kidding around, his mood lightened a bit as he continued. "That stunt you pulled back at the bar got the cops involved, bro. I barely made it out before they arrived. Why the hell did you throw that mug at the bouncer?"

Suddenly the memory came flooding back. I remembered meeting up with a girl and buying her a drink. I also remembered hearing the people sitting next to us talking about me. I could still remember feeling their eyes on me, staring and judging. What I had heard, or thought I heard, had ticked me off. As at every juncture in my life, I didn't think: I lashed out.

Though unable to recall every detail, I remembered approaching the men at the next table and pushing the first one who met my gaze. As the exchange quickly exploded, I remember holding a thick beer mug in my hand and chucking it across the bar, missing the bartender by inches. The glass shattered against the wall, and the bouncers and staff closed in on me. I remembered wanting to fight, but luckily Mike had taken action, pushing toward the door and shouting for me to run. Feeling like everyone in the club was out to get me, I wasn't about to be captured. Shoving my way through the chaos, I barely made it out the door before breaking into a full run.

Thinking about it, I couldn't help but chuckle, which Mike did not appreciate. Pushing me, he spoke with a harsh tone, although he was having a hard time not smiling. "Seriously, bro, you could've gotten me busted, especially with the crap I'm holding for you."

When Mike pushed me, I could feel my temper flare up. I almost lashed out, but I was distracted by the sound of laughter. We were getting closer to the clubs. Interested in getting back to the clubs, I shrugged. "How about I buy you a round? We'll forget what happened and have some fun."

"Are you nuts?" Mike shook his head, holding me back. "You can't go back there, bro. Not for a few weeks. Besides, it's three in the morning, and the clubs aren't serving alcohol."

"Doesn't mean we can't have some fun," I responded as I pointed at Mike's pocket, which was filled with illicit drugs.

"You are a bad influence," Mike said with a chuckle as he pointed to my sleeve. He was no stranger to trouble, and I think he found my sudden explosions entertaining. "If that sleeve hadn't ripped, you'd be sitting in jail right now. I still can't believe you broke that bouncer's grip."

Finally knowing how my arm had been scratched and my shirt torn, I shrugged. I should have been asking questions or wondering why I had lashed out with such violence, but all I could focus on was how to extend the evening. As usual, I was focused only on myself and pleasure, unaware and uncaring of my actions or the potential consequences. Although I was drunk and drugged and should've been tired, my mind was racing, and I was filled with an immense amount of energy that I was itching to burn off.

"We can still hit a few after-hours clubs," Mike suggested, making my wild eyes flash with excitement. In Denver, last call didn't make the night scene vanish; it just changed. The after-hours clubs were a place for drugs and a more extreme approach to partying. Although the after-hours clubs tried to police their establishments, there was just no way to control every individual.

"Sounds good to me," I said. I always enjoyed partying with Mike. He was one of my more radical friends and went out with me when my other friends were avoiding me. This was mostly because he found me entertaining, but it was also due to the fact that his drug and alcohol problems made him less sensitive to my sudden outbursts and explosions. I didn't know it at the time, but my erratic behavior had already begun to terrify my closest friends and family.

I lived at home in my parents' basement and was in college, which wouldn't last for long. Every aspect of my life was unstable, and I was unable to hold down a job or maintain any relationship, professional or personal. Mike was one of the few friends who stuck by me. Although Mike was just my party friend, unconnected to me in any other way, even he was sometimes caught off guard by my sudden outbursts of violence or radical mood swings. It would be years later that Mike would vanish, lost to the drugs he always longed for.

After we spent three more hours at an after-hours club, the sun was up, and Mike was ready to go. Sober now, I was still aching for more action. My mind was continuing to speed from one thought to another, and I was having a hard time concentrating. We had run out of drugs, so we ended the night, even with my objections.

The drive home was quick, and I was enjoying the feel of his car on the highway. "Dude, you gotta slow down. And would you please stop talking? My head is killing me."

Mike's hangover had finally caught up to him. A bit ticked off that he had told me to quiet down, I cranked up the radio and pushed his car above ninety miles an hour. Mike sighed, knowing me well enough to understand that I wasn't going to listen. When I arrived home, it was seven in the morning, and I wasn't the least bit tired. "How about tonight?"

Mike looked at me like I was crazy. "Dude, don't you sleep?" Mike chuckled, seeing that I wasn't kidding as he added, "We'll see."

I moved out of the way so Mike could get into the driver's seat. "Just plan on tonight. It'll be fun."

"It's always an adventure," Mike said before closing the door and driving out of the cul-de-sac.

I stood there for a moment, alone in my parents' driveway. What I didn't know at the time was that my manic episodes were not a single-stage event. They always started off with a sudden spike of energy and productivity until I reached a second stage, during which my focus was lost and all I wanted to do was slow my mind down.

Standing in the driveway, I could feel that stage giving way to what I can only describe as a third stage, or a peak. Although I didn't know it at the time, this third and final stage was always accompanied by delusions of grandiosity. It was also accompanied by paranoia, thinking that someone might steal my great ideas or that everyone was conspiring against me. That mixture made for a dangerous combination, leading me to start more fights than I can recall. Luckily, I had never been seriously injured nor done so to another, not because I wasn't trying but because I usually started fights with multiple individuals. I took quite a few beatings throughout the years.

Although many of the most inspired, productive, and creative moments in my life came when I was at the first stage of my mania, the price I paid for those flashes of brilliance was never worth the cost. My manic peaks would end with a terrifying eruption of violence and anger that made me a danger to myself and everyone around me. I wouldn't know until years later that that peak was a warning that I was about to crash into a deep depression. It never failed. The higher and more intense the peak, the quicker and more violent the fall into darkness.

II.   MANIA'S RAZOR EDGE

As I stood in the driveway, the sun continued to rise above the Denver skyline, beginning to cast its warm glow onto our small street and my mother's garden. When I entered the house at around seven thirty, I found my mother and father standing in the kitchen staring at me, deep circles under their eyes. Their worry quickly turned to flashes of anger, and I became defensive and prepared for a fight. They were both gentle and kind people, but they were growing tired of my radical emotions.

"Where have you been?" my mother asked. "I've been worried sick. The least you could've done was call." Unlike the people who knew me only as a friend, those who lived with me saw the truth and severity of my mental state. They were aware of exactly how violent and irrational I could become.

I didn't care about my mother's concern as my mania was quickly rising beyond my control. "I'm twenty-one years old, Mom," I lashed out in a harsh voice. "You can cut the parent crap!" My mother took a step back, a bit of surprise edging out the anger on her face as my dad stood up and stepped between us.

"That's no way to talk to your mother."

I was taller and more muscular than my father, and when I walked past I slammed my shoulder into him in an act that still repulses me. As I had my entire life, I saw everyone as two extremes: friend or enemy. At the moment I didn't see my parents but just people out to criticize and judge me. "Lay off!" I shouted at them as I walked toward the basement door. "I was out with friends."

I had been in a great mood, but my jubilation had quickly transformed into an anger that I couldn't shake. In a final show of rage, I took hold of the door, slamming it shut as I walked into the basement. The force I had put on the door broke the handle and caused the door to crack. Too furious to go to bed and unable to focus, I decided I would paint.

Handling my mania was like walking on a razor's edge. I didn't understand anything about my mind or what was wrong at the time, nor did I realize that I was becoming more dangerous, angry, violent, paranoid, and delusional. With no ability to analyze myself, I was trapped between euphoria and utter despair. The only thing keeping my mind from crashing was the paint that I was hastily and violently stroking onto the canvas.

I had no way of knowing that my mania was going to grow more intense and eventually peak. I didn't even know what mania was. It is easy now to understand that the first stage of my mania made me witty, playful, and confident. I loved those moments; I was always productive, and going out with my usual friends was extremely fun. It was the following stages that always spiraled out of control and caused damage to my relationships and life. It was typically during the second stage that I would go out drinking and seeking any and all drugs in an attempt to calm and quiet my mind.

Currently, my second stage was quickly speeding out of control.

Even as I painted, I couldn't shake my anger. Anger, aggressiveness, and frustration with everything around me were clues that I was about to hit my peak. Unfortunately for me and the people I cared for, the others around me did not know about my mental state and were always surprised at my sudden outbursts of violent speech, actions, and anger at the world and everyone in it.

Even the way I handled the brushes was violent. The strokes of paint were not thought out, just actions; I believed I was meant for greater things than the average person. I broke two brushes just because they had not delivered the effect I was looking for. Slowly, the anger in me was bubbling up, but there was nothing to trigger it. I was a ticking bomb, just waiting to be set off. As I finished one painting, I set it down, staring at it with a heightened sense of pride that led me to wonder why I was not yet famous. Painting faster, I had no idea that I had been at it for six straight hours with no sleep and no food. In the end, I had painted four large landscapes.

It was during these peaks that I became delusional enough to believe I was capable of anything, believing that the world was lucky to have me and that fame would soon be knocking at my door. I had no idea that these peaks were a warning of a coming depression where I would feel as though even breathing wasn't worth my time.

Looking proudly at my paintings, my mind was racing with thoughts of fame and riches. My book was going to be a bestseller, and my paintings would make me millions, not to mention that I had figured out the secret to trading stocks. I certainly was beyond anything that I could learn at college or a job. Of course, I was mistaken.

Hearing my sister come into the house, I took hold of the largest of the paintings. I hadn't gotten anything for her birthday, but what could be better than an original painting by her soon-to-be-famous brother. When I got upstairs, I presented the painting to my family that had been so worried about me. Like always, everyone wasn't sure what mood I would be in, but they were glad that I was not shouting. Before my sister saw the painting, I could see that she had heard that I had gotten back late and had worried my parents, but she quickly averted her gaze and focused on the painting. Everyone loved what I had painted for my sister, but I could sense that they were still upset.

"Kirk," my sister said cautiously and quietly, as if she wasn't sure she should say anything. Slowly, she pointed to my cargo shorts and the streaks of paint that stained them. "Your favorite shorts. Why don't we get those into the wash …"

I had forgotten to change before painting, but my sister's voice trailed off as I looked down at the stains. It was such a small thing, but apparently my sister and parents could see the impending explosion. All three took a step back.

Staring at the stains, all positive feelings I might have felt were swept away, and my mania entered the third and most volatile stage. At first my voice was quiet, although my knuckles were turning white as I gripped the edge of the painting. "Son of a—" I didn't finish my statement before turning around and punching the door to the basement as hard as I could. Although the door wasn't solid core, it didn't break with the first hit but instead cracked down the middle. I had already damaged the door earlier and was angry that I hadn't shattered it. The violence and suddenness of my action made my family jump, and I noticed my sister jerk back in surprise.

"Kirken," my sister said gently, always the peacekeeper, "I'm sure Mom can get the stains out."

"No!" I shouted, feeling my mind spinning out of control. Assuming that everyone in the world was against me, I pointed toward the stains as if my sister couldn't see them. "This is oil paint. They're ruined!" Cursing, I tore my shorts off, stripping down to my boxers before slamming my fist into anything nearby. Punching multiple holes in the drywall as I stormed out to the garage, I could hear my mother and sister crying as my dad shouted for me to calm down. I was lost to them, their voices like a whisper in a hurricane.

Overrun by the river of rage that was flooding my every fiber, I left the kitchen and walked through the garage, walking down the driveway toward my car. Wanting to lash out at everything, rage overwhelming my every sense, I punched the mailbox until it flew off its wooden stand. I had no idea that my hand was bruised and bleeding as my family rushed out, worried about me driving in my current state.

My sister's pleading was of no use, and I was beyond being reached by words or actions as I entered the driver's seat, starting the engine. Suddenly aware that my storm of curse words and actions had drawn the attention of our neighbors, I felt like I was being watched as if I were a rabid dog. I think it was out of fear that no one called the police, yet I didn't care as I closed and locked the driver's-side door before ripping out of the cul-de-sac. I couldn't be contained or calmed, and I hate to think of what I might have done had the police shown up to detain me.

My tires squealed as I flew through the gentle neighborhood, my foot pressed down on the gas pedal as I remember wondering: *Why am I even here?* At that moment, I truly hated myself and the world. Seeping in self-pity, I couldn't see beyond myself. I didn't worry about my family or how I had verbally attacked the very people who loved me. I didn't even see them as family members, but as enemies who were plotting against me.

Eventually I slowed down and pulled off to the side of the road. My mind was quickly shutting down. The colors around me seemed dull and gray, like the fog of depression that was quickly overtaking me. Even the anger that had been driving me had vanished, leaving me wondering if I should simply drive off a cliff and end my suffering.

Pulling the emergency brake and shifting into neutral, I rested my forehead on the steering wheel. I wanted to shout out or cry, but I had stopped crying by the time I was in third grade. The mania that had been protecting me from the pain that was now throbbing from my bloody and swollen knuckles and bare feet was gone, but the physical pain was nothing compared to the mental anguish that had suddenly cast a shadow over my entire worldview. In a few short moments, I had gone from feeling capable of fame and fortune to a sense of worthlessness, vulnerability, hopelessness, and self-loathing.

III. SHATTERED MANIA AND THE FALL INTO DESPAIR

I sat in the car for a long time, my body feeling heavy. My lips tightened as I tried hard to breathe, but I felt as though a heavy blanket had been draped over me. Not only was it hard to breathe but I also wasn't sure if I cared. With my head and hands resting on the steering wheel, dressed only in a T-shirt and boxers, I didn't care about anything.

The radio was on, but the music sounded distant. My throbbing hands and feet seemed disconnected, and I wasn't aware of the damage

I had caused, nor could I feel any pain. The darkness that was draped over my mind dulled everything and distorted time. Not having any place to go and nowhere I desired to be, I just sat there, unmoving and uncaring. I wondered what it would be like if I simply fell asleep and never woke up. My mania had peaked, and I had crashed down into a pool of self-loathing. Although I had been a completely different person during the previous three weeks as my mania had been ramping up, I didn't know anything was wrong. All my life, I had been unpredictable. From a very young age, I was impossible to discipline as I simply didn't care, nor did I see the same reality that others did. The inability to understand reality would become worse with each passing year, until I was less human than beast at the age of twenty-one or twenty-two.

Looking back, it is clear that I had been overcome with a heavy depression, but at the time, I didn't even know or care that I had been a completely different person only hours ago. To change so drastically was something I should have noticed, but my mind was simply unaware of anything but what I was feeling at the moment. In fact, everything good that had ever happened to me seemed like a façade. It was as if someone had tricked me into believing in happiness.

Tired of the blaring music, I began to reach forward to turn off the radio and was surprised at how hard such a simple motion was. My arm felt heavy, and the desire to move simply wasn't strong enough, so I left the radio on as the music stopped and advertisements blared out of the speakers. Dropping my arm down just before I reached the radio's control, I gave up on everything.

Tired of everything, including my life, I wanted to shout toward the heavens and curse whatever force had brought me into existence, but even the idea of shouting seemed overwhelming. I should've been surprised when I heard someone tapping their knuckles against my window, but I didn't even move my head.

When my door was opened from the outside and I felt a hand gently touch my shoulder, I didn't even move. Had it been a few hours earlier, I might have snapped, but I was devoid of energy and didn't want to open my eyes. When my sister spoke, her voice seemed distant yet gentle. "Are you hurt? Did something happen?"

I didn't answer.

"I'm going to take you home, okay?" my sister said, asking permission as she took hold of my left arm and gently pulled, trying to help me out of the driver's seat. My body felt heavy, and although I didn't want to see or talk to anyone, I didn't have the energy to fight, so I let my sister guide me around the back of the car and into the passenger's seat. Plopping down in the seat, I didn't even reach out to close the door.

"Can you get the door?" my sister asked before walking away. Her voice was laced with frustration but mostly concern. When I was unable to move, my sister made sure the door wouldn't hit me and closed it before walking around to the driver's side.

After the door shut, I leaned my head against the cool glass, staring into the rearview mirror and recognizing my father's headlights. As always, I was lost in my own reality, feeling unloved by the world and the people close to me. Even as I was being taken care of, I was unable to comprehend that my family had cared enough to come looking for me.

When my sister got into the car, she turned off the stereo and pointed to my seat belt. "Put your seat belt on." I didn't move, keeping my head against the window. My mind was so foggy that although I had heard her suggestion, I couldn't respond. Like the amazing sister she was, Chandi reached over, took hold of my seat belt, and buckled me in. After clicking me safely into place, my sister continued to talk. "Did you hit something? Why were you just sitting there on the side of the road?"

For the first time I spoke. "Does it really matter?" I responded, my voice flat and hollow.

"Of course it does," my sister said gently as if she were trying to soothe me. I didn't notice. I was unable to think of anything other than how horrible my life was even though, in reality, I was very blessed and loved.

"What were you thinking?" Chandi asked, sighing as she added, "You realize you owe everyone an apology. You had everyone worried sick, and you certainly did a good job getting the neighbors' attention."

"Like it matters," was all I could say. "I just want to sleep." The statement was only half-true. I did want to sleep, but I didn't want to wake up to the world that had turned on me and that felt so strange and bleak.

Like much of my past, I wasn't aware of what was happening. It is only now that I realize that my mind had shut down. The mania had vanished from beneath my feet, leaving me to fall into the beginning of my depressive phase. Much like my mania, my depression also had different stages. My first stage of depression would make my mind feel sluggish, and I was always left with the feeling that everything I had been working for either was slipping away or was already gone. It was also a time when I stayed away from my friends and family. Actually, I stayed away from anything that I enjoyed, even though I needed support, joy, and love more than ever during those times.

Most people only saw my first stage of mania, in which I was pleasant, witty, and upbeat. This masked my mental disability from even those who knew me best. My closest friends and relatives had no idea how much I was suffering or the pain I caused my family, while those unlucky enough to live with me saw the darkest sides of my swings.

Many people blamed teenage hormones for my swings. As the years went by, however, my moods became more severe and disruptive. But I had always been out of control, and even when I was a child my reactions were out of touch with reality. Drugs and alcohol did not help, but they certainly didn't cause the bipolar that plagued me. Looking back makes it clear that bipolar had always ruled my life. As I grew older my swings began to worry my family, as they not only disrupted every aspect of my own life but took a heavy and devastating toll on those dearest to me.

When we arrived home, I got out of the car before anyone could speak to me. It took all of my energy just to push open my door, stand up, and walk into the house. As I stepped into the kitchen, my head down, my shoulders slumped forward, and my boxers twisted, I felt that I deserved to be punished, almost wishing God would strike me down. When no flash of lightening came to end what I felt was a pathetic life, I headed into my basement, closing the door and collapsing on my bed.

Closing my eyes, I was unable to escape the feeling that I was trapped by some unseen force. As if a heavy weight were pressing down on my chest, my breathing was shallow, my eyes were sensitive, and I welcomed death. Make no mistake, I never wanted to feel so depressed, but the harder I tried to climb out of the depression that had overtaken me, the tighter the cage that held me in darkness became.

I just need to sleep, I remember thinking, completely unaware that the anguish I felt was only the beginning stage of my depressive swing and was only going to get worse.

IV. DEEPENING DEPRESSION

I awoke the next day feeling no different than the night before. Not only did I not want to get up, but I hated the fact that I had awakened. All I wanted was to sleep, but my depression was still in the first stage. I was slightly hungry, and, since I hadn't showered in two days, I smelled.

Getting out of bed took nearly an hour and more energy than I thought I could muster. Unable to hold a steady job or stay in college, I remember focusing on how messed up the world was. I hated the idea that every day felt the same as I struggled to gain a foothold on my dreams. When I analyze myself now, I can't help but see that I was always focused on dreams and not my future. Everything was based on the present, with no ability to sense or fear my past or future, making my depressions torturous. The inability to see beyond the moment might be considered a good thing to some, but without reality to ground me, it was beyond a hindrance.

I know now that having even a slight grasp of what I wanted in the future would've helped guide my present, but my logical skills were lost in depression and tainted to an extreme during my manias. Although I had dreams like anyone else, my inability to focus on how to reach my lofty goals made me miss out on the steps I needed to take in order to make my dreams and goals a reality. Believing that I was too smart and too important for school or work when I was manic made me dismiss opportunities during my depression stages. My goals felt impossible, and I did not really care if I reached them or not.

Going to the bathroom, I just sat on the floor, wondering why I had to suffer. What god would cause such pain, and what had I done to deserve such a fate?

Eventually I stood up and walked back to my room. It was summer break, not that it mattered. College had already proven too steady and regimented for me to handle. Although I had started strong, my transcripts showed my swings. One semester I would take on too many credits, and the next I would take the minimum class load. Eventually I dropped out of college, falling back on the only skill I had, playing the violin to make a few dollars when I could. After giving up a full-tuition scholarship at the University of Denver because I had seen a rainbow that I had believed was a sign that I should follow my dreams of writing, painting, and fame, all I had was my skill with the violin. Unable to handle teaching violin students in my current state, I could still play at weddings and events when not depressed.

Standing up slowly, I entered my small basement shower, welcoming the pain of water slamming into the cuts on my arm and fists. My hand was swollen and black from hitting everything in sight, but the disturbing part was that I felt I deserved to feel pain. Glancing at the razor in the shower, I picked it up, slowly turning it in my hand. I stared at the polished steel blades while wondering if I should end it all.

Sighing, I didn't even have the drive to shave or soap my body down, let alone end my life. Putting the blade back up, I turned off the water and walked out of the shower and into my room. I didn't even dry off or close the shower door as I walked into my room, naked.

On my dresser was a napkin from the previous night with a woman's phone number written in blue ink. Next to the note was a new pair of the same shorts I had ruined the night before, but I didn't even care that my mom had not only taken the time to find another pair but spent her own money in an attempt to cheer me up. The idea of calling anyone sounded like torture, so I crawled into bed, not even bothering to dry or dress myself.

As I closed my eyes, I knew that I wanted nothing to do with anything, anyone, or the world. I wasn't happy, but every time I thought of something that might make me feel better, my chest tightened and I felt a heavy wave of sadness that kept my mind from even thinking about anything pleasurable. *This isn't what life is supposed to be,* I thought as I fell asleep, unaware that a few tears had fallen out of the corner of my eyes, rolling down my chin and falling to my pillow.

I didn't improve over the next two weeks, and every day I struggled just to keep moving. I didn't understand why I even tried to shower or eat, as the only time I felt any break from a feeling of worthlessness was when I slept. I had been able to teach, since I only had three students at the time, all of whom I liked, but with each passing day everything became more strenuous and stressful.

My family tried to talk to me and help, but the conversations were brief. I was easily agitated, making my family tense and worried. It was clear that my mother and sister were trying to cheer me up, but whenever they tried I turned cold and quickly retreated to the safety of my dark basement. I wanted to feel better, but I had no way of climbing out of the dark abyss I was in. Worst of all, I was completely unaware that anything was wrong with me. All my life, bipolar was there, affecting me and my relationships. At the age of ten I was diagnosed with ADHD, but at that time bipolar wasn't something anyone was looking for.

In my opinion, it was the world that was tainted, and I wanted no part of it. In many ways, this lack of reality protected me from seeing the truth. Had I been aware of all the relationships I had ruined, I have no doubt that I would've taken my own life.

After two weeks of depression, I still felt no relief, and each day felt worse and darker than the previous one. The only thing that was changing was the intensity with which I hated myself. I didn't want to feel down, but nothing worked to lighten my mood. I was unable to function on the most basic level, so playing video games, going out, watching a movie, lifting at the gym, or hanging out with friends were impossible to fathom. Therefore, I had spent the past two weeks in my basement, coming out only to use the bathroom.

When the third week came, my depression grew darker, and I was unable to answer phone calls, shower, or even eat. My mother and sister did their best to act like nothing was wrong and smile when around me, but I could see through their facades. My dad just looked worried. In many ways, my bipolar stayed hidden for as long as it did because I never let anyone but my family see my downs. It wasn't that I knew that I was depressed and was trying to hide it. I simply didn't want to and couldn't handle seeing anyone.

When looking back, my family feels foolish that they didn't realize how deeply disturbed I was, but none of the therapists my mother had taken me to had caught it either. Not only is bipolar hard to diagnose but it stays hidden until it begins to rip your life apart. I just feel lucky that they loved me and did take actions once things grew worse.

Staying in my room and sleeping the days away, I wanted the pain to go away, but it was out of my control. As a gentle knock sounded against my door, I rolled over and faced the wall. I didn't want to see anyone, but I hadn't locked my room and wasn't about to move.

My mom's voice sounded soft and gentle as she spoke, "Kirk, can I come in?" I didn't answer as she slowly opened the door. Seeing that I was facing the wall, she shook a plastic bag that she had brought into my room. Even the sound of the bag seemed overwhelming as my mother said, "I thought you might be hungry, so I went out and picked you up a sandwich. It's your favorite."

"Thanks," I said in a whisper. Talking was quickly becoming harder for me as I grew more distant and depressed with each passing day. Constant thoughts of suicide bombarded me, and I was unable to stop picturing or thinking about ending my life. However, as much as I wanted to end my suffering, I simply wasn't able to shake off the heavy blanket of anguish to act on any of my darker thoughts. The depression that had ensnared me felt like it was getting tighter, slowly squeezing the life out of me. In truth, I just assumed that I was going to die.

Setting a Subway sandwich down on my dresser, my mom came to my side. She sat down next to me and leaned over to give me a hug in an attempt to comfort me. I tensed up and pushed her away. My mind was lost enough that the only thing working were my instincts. I didn't even realize that all I wanted was a gentle hug, nor could I communicate such a desire. My mom's attempt was sweet, but the physical touch felt overwhelming and strangely foreign.

It would have helped to have someone just sitting quietly on the floor beside me, but I could neither recognize my needs nor verbalize them. When I pulled away, my mother knew there was nothing she could do, so she stood up, left the food on my dresser, and quietly exited my room. Unable to see beyond my own twisted and bleak reality, I was always unaware of the people around me. It was not an easy life for me, but at times it was harder on those who loved me.

I never ate the sandwich, as I felt no hunger. Trying to avoid the pain that was suffocating me, I retreated into a deep sleep. The second stage of my depression had come and gone, and the third and final stage hit me hard. The last thought before sleep took me away was wishing death would take me because I was unable to take my own life.

That weekend I couldn't eat or move from my bed other than to go to the bathroom. I hadn't shaved or showered in a week and had lost enough weight to look a bit sick. Although my parents and sister tried to get me moving, I refused any help. Although I was in a weakened state, I was unstable enough and strong enough that my parents and sister couldn't help. The only thing they could do was call a mental institution, but I believe they couldn't accept just how bad I was. Had they known that all I wanted was to die and that the only thing keeping me from ending my life was the effort it would take, they would've taken much more drastic steps. In many ways, it was my inability to function that kept me safe from suicide. Had I been able to move or function, I have no doubt that I would've acted on my darkest thoughts.

The next time I woke up was because my room's lights had been flicked on. The harsh light was an attack on my senses. When my eyes fluttered open, my vision was blurry, and I felt confused. Although I couldn't rate how bad I had felt before falling asleep, I knew, without a doubt, that I was far worse than before. Even talking seemed like an impossible feat. Walking to the side of my bed, my sister gently touched my forearm and spoke firmly. "It's Monday, and you've been sleeping for nearly two days." My sister was tired of my behavior and pulled back my sheets before continuing her motherly speech. "You need to get up and stop acting like a child."

I tried to respond, but my voice never came, and I was unable to move or think. My sister was home alone and unaware of my mental state. Had my parents been there, seeing me in that state, they might have taken action and called for help. My sister, however, was determined to do her best to look after me. Only now do I understand how lucky I was to have Chandi in my life. Seeing frustration bloom on my sister's face, I closed my eyes again. Everything about my reality was overwhelming, making me feel out of place and lost.

"You haven't eaten in three days, and you smell," Chandi said, taking hold of my arm as she tried to get me moving. "Kirk," she shouted when she was unable to move me. I wasn't fighting her. I just wasn't moving and was far too large for Chandi's small stature to move. "You need to get up and get cleaned up. Come on!" After giving my arm one last tug, my sister finally gave up. My arm fell limply back to the bed. My sister waited for me to respond, but I failed to move. I could hear her crying as she turned and walked out my room, turning the light off before closing the door behind her.

Alone again, I tried to speak, but even opening my mouth felt like an overwhelming feat of strength. My mind was no longer functioning as I lay there, trying to breathe. Suicide was now far too complicated for my fuddled mind to handle. If I couldn't speak, shower, shave, eat, or move, I certainly wasn't able to take my own life. Therefore, I closed my eyes again, screaming inside but unable to voice my pain.

For two more weeks I was unable to break through the cage of depression that continued to tighten around me. I had been bad before, but this was the first time I hadn't been able to move or talk. After three weeks of my worst depression yet, my mother came into my room. Even without the light turned on, it was easy to see that her face was somber as she sat down beside me.

"Kirk, I think you need help." Had I cared about anything or been able to think, I'm sure I would have denied my mom's hypothesis, but I was lost in the overwhelming pain I felt. I just wanted the suffering to stop. "I called the doctor, and he gave me the name of a good psychiatrist. The soonest I could get us into see him was in two weeks. I know we've seen psychologists in the past, but I can't do this anymore. We need to try again."

Leaving me with her words, my mother stood up and left the room. Even then, unable to eat, move, or care about anything, I didn't realize anything was wrong. I was sure that it was the world that was twisted and not my mind.

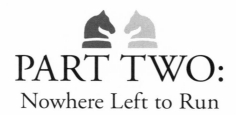

PART TWO:
Nowhere Left to Run

:: Seeking Help Even When the Truth Hurts ::

I.   SEEKING HELP

It doesn't take long when looking back at my life and my behavior to realize how lucky I am to still be alive. I wouldn't be had my family not known that I was beyond helping myself. Although I had seen psychologists in my youth, it was because I was always acting out and explosive. When my mother made an appointment with one of the leading psychiatrists in Colorado, I figured it would be the same dance all over again. This time, however, was different. I wasn't seeing a psychiatrist because I was in need of some simple guidance. This time, I was seeing a specialist because my family had run out of options and believed something was truly wrong with me. Although I had been bipolar my entire life, the previous two years had grown out of control, leaving my parents no option but to face the idea that something was truly wrong with me.

I admit I was desperately in need of help, but at the time I thought I was fine. I actually felt betrayed by those who were supposed to love me the most for even thinking something might be wrong with me. Truly believing I was just having a rough time, I couldn't see or understand just how serious of a risk I was to myself and others. Even had the bipolar not blurred my vision of reality, no one wants to believe there is something wrong, and I was no exception. I didn't like seeing a doctor for a cough, but I despised the idea of seeing a specialist when the sole purpose was to determine my sanity. Although I didn't want to waste my time seeing another therapist, I was still trapped in my depression, and I didn't have the energy to fight or run. When the time came, I reluctantly got into the car with my mom, and we drove off to meet a top psychiatrist whom I will refer to as Dr. Smith. Although the worst of my depression had faded, I was still irritable, and moving or leaving was quite difficult for me.

During the drive I sat quietly in the car, staring out the window as we drove by a run-down amusement park that was on the way to Dr. Smith's office. When the tall buildings started rising into the sky around us, I knew we were getting close. I did not want to speak to anyone, and I certainly didn't feel like speaking to a psychiatrist. However, I didn't have the energy to fight with my mother about the merits of seeing the psychiatrist or expressing that I thought it was a waste of time.

Turning into a large parking lot filled with an immense gray stone building that blocked the sun and cast a long shadow across the cars and street, my mom parked the car, turned off the radio, and turned to face me.

"Thank you for trying this, honey," my mother said, looking over at me with her warm blue eyes, which were filled with worry.

I nodded as I slowly opened the door. Although the worst of my depression was fading, I walked across the parking lot hunched over, my head down and my eyes focused on the ground. My posture changed depending on my moods, and analyzing old pictures shows that my eyes were dull and empty when I was down and brilliant and wild when I was manic.

Following my mom as if there were an invisible chain she was pulling me with, I had no idea how I looked or felt and was convinced I was fine. I didn't want to waste my time or my parents' money to hear what I already knew. Had I not been recovering from my worst depression ever, I would've fought seeing a specialist with every ounce of my strength.

The two glass doors that stood at the entrance to the building were heavy. We walked into a large marble entryway. To my left there was a bank, and to my right were two elevators that I wasn't looking forward to entering. I knew that if I had more energy I wouldn't have gotten onto the elevator.

"Come on." My mother took hold of my arm with a gentle grip, guiding me onto the elevator. There was another woman on the elevator who looked at me with what felt like caution, her eyes quickly seeing my hunched posture and my dull eyes. I quickly noticed that she was looking at me and stared back. I didn't understand why the woman with straight brown hair and hazel eyes was staring at me, but I didn't like it. After a long and intense glare, she looked away and down at the floor. Sensing the tension, my mother pulled me to the back of the elevator, pressing a button while making small talk with the woman in an attempt to cut the tension. Often I would feel that people were staring at me, judging me, and, at my manic peaks, plotting against me.

What makes my feelings so hypocritical is how I always judged others without a second glance. Looking back, it is appalling to realize how quickly I decided if someone was a friend or foe. Like my emotions, there were only extremes and no room for a middle ground. Good friendships and relationships were ruined because of the tricks my mind and moods played on me. When I was manic or depressed, my view of life and everything in it was twisted, always leading me to act out in ways that were far beyond reason.

In the rare moments when I was between mania and depression I did have a good sense of people; however, those moments were both rare and fleeting. This made relationships, both personal and professional, nearly impossible to nurture. Relationships are hard enough when one is thinking clearly and calmly, but the reality I observed through my bipolar eyes was never calm and often warped. Because of this, I pushed people away and always ended up alone.

My warped worldview affected my life in many ways other than just my relationships. In fact, many of my major life decisions were made after paranoia, anger, mistrust, and delusions led me to form false conclusions. What baffles me is how dedicated I was to my worldview. If I decided I wouldn't like something, there was not a force strong enough to change my mind. The same was true with what I liked.

When I was lost in the depths of a manic or depressive swing, the decisions I made, logical or not, were carved in stone. I would make rash decisions or come to a radical conclusion that others saw as comical, strange, or horrific. No matter how large or drastic my decisions were, once my mind was made up, I was committed deeply to the decisions I made and never thought twice about my resulting actions. This went for people, art, clothing, food, schoolwork, music, and pretty much everything in life.

As usual, I had already made my decision about the woman who had briefly met my eyes. I didn't like her. Looking away from the woman, I stared into the mirrors that lined the elevator and rested on a polished marble base. Instead of noticing the beauty of the elevator, all I could focus on were the fingerprints and smears on the polished surfaces.

When the elevator began to move, I continued to stick to the idea that seeing a shrink was a waste of time. I hated change, something I have found to be very common in others suffering from bipolar. When the door opened and the woman stepped off, I said in a harsh and sarcastic voice, "Have a nice day, ma'am." Whether I was manic or lightly depressed, I was often very aggressive. Clearly, the woman had done nothing wrong. I felt satisfaction when she quickened her pace, until I noticed my mother's stare.

"What?" I exclaimed, "She was giving me a nasty look for no reason."

"I thought you promised me you would give this a try." My mother's tone was serious as she looked at me. "You gave me your word."

Although there was not much that remained steady in my life, I did have a strong sense of honor, and when I gave my word, I tried my best to keep it. The only times I ever broke my word were when I was at the peak stage of either depression or mania. Of course, I was never aware that I had broken my word, but now, as I analyze my past with a clear and balanced mind, I see how fickle even my honor was.

"Fine," I said, pulling myself away and crossing my arms defiantly. I would keep my word. "Sorry," I added without any sincerity.

The elevator stopped and made an annoying dinging sound as the doors slid open. "Here we are," my mother said, offering a gentle smile as she stepped off and walked to the wall directly across from the elevators. I reluctantly followed, staring at the list of names and office numbers my mother was checking. "This won't take long. Just remember that you promised me you would cooperate."

I huffed as I followed her. My favorite yellow jacket was too warm for the weather, but I didn't really notice. My mind was focused on the doors as we passed by. I didn't feel any apprehension as the office numbers grew closer to our destination and certainly didn't have enough energy to resist.

Dr. Smith's office was at the end of the hallway. He was a highly regarded psychiatrist who had been suggested to us by multiple doctors, but I wasn't sold. When my mom opened the heavy wooden door to Dr. Smith's office, I paused for a split second before entering the waiting room.

Walking over to the couches that encircled a nice table filled with magazines, I plopped down and grabbed a random magazine as my mom checked me in and filled out the paperwork. It's sad for me to think that my mom even had to fill out my papers, but I was never very cooperative when it came to something I didn't agree with.

After my mom finished with the paperwork she handed it to the nurse, who I thought seemed extremely grumpy. The nurse pressed a small red button on the wall before speaking, "Mrs. Miller, Dr. Smith will be right with you. Just sit down and make yourself comfortable."

When the door opened, a man stepped forward. Dressed in a maroon sweater, nice slacks, and polished wing-tip shoes that looked expensive, he looked briefly at the receptionist and then in my direction. His head was bald except for the slightly curly gray hair sticking out beyond his ears and resting low on his hawk-nose was a pair of thin, rectangular glasses. He looked like they had pulled a psychiatrist out of the movies to play his part. Looking over the edges of his glasses, he met my eyes. "Kirk, I presume?" Although he spoke quietly, his voice felt cold to me. Turning to my mother, he smiled and shook her hand. "And you must be Jeanne."

As my mother nodded, he added, "It is nice to meet you both" before leading us down the hallway and opening the door to his corner office. Gesturing toward the leather chairs and sofas, Dr. Smith smiled and said, "Please, sit down and make yourselves comfortable."

I sat down on the soft leather couch, and my mother sat next to me. Dr. Smith pulled out a yellow legal pad and pen along with a file that must have come from the other doctors and psychologists I had seen over the years. Unlike when I went to see a psychologist, this wasn't to work on family or school problems. This time, I was suddenly becoming aware that it was my sanity that was being evaluated. I didn't feel fear, for I knew I was fine. I had no idea that my entire life was about to change.

II.   DIAGNOSIS AND DISBELIEF

Once we were all seated, Dr. Smith quickly explained that before he could come to any conclusions or diagnosis, he first had to ensure that my behavior was not the direct result of any medical issues, medications, or illicit drugs that could cause some of the same symptoms found in mental disorders. Luckily, our family doctor had made sure that the psychiatrist had all the medical information Dr. Smith needed.

After seeing that we both understood, Dr. Smith sat down in an expensive-looking chair that sat opposite us and in front of his antique wooden desk. Leaning back, Dr. Smith lifted a thick manila folder resting on his desk. I stared at the folder, knowing that the file contained all the information the doctors and psychologists had gathered. Everything from my medical tests and psychological tests was held within the folder. A part of me wanted to see what the other psychologists had written, but I quickly lost interest. If all I had to do was put up with one more doctor and his questions to prove once and for all that I was sound of mind, I was okay with that.

Dr. Smith crossed his legs, carefully scanning the file that he had already marked and flagged. For a few minutes, we sat in silence as Dr. Smith proved that he was just as meticulous and cautious as we had been told. To me, he felt cold and calculating, but I wasn't happy about anything that morning and was looking for any excuse to dismiss anything the man said.

Keeping his eyes on the file, Dr. Smith suddenly spoke. "Do you mind if I ask you some questions?"

I remember sighing. I had been through this before and wasn't looking forward to answering the same questions that all the other mental professionals had asked. To my surprise, his questions were very different than what I was expecting. Most of the questions were very simple, requiring little time for me to give my cold response, such as whether I cried and how often. Did I ever hear sounds or see things that others didn't? The questions kept coming, but after about ten minutes the questions became more obscure. I don't remember most of them as they seemed so simple at the time. What surprised me was that some were easy to answer and others required time to contemplate. Watching the doctor pause occasionally before asking another question, I found myself growing curious about what he was writing about me. Suddenly, however, his questions became very detailed.

"I notice that you dropped out of college. It looks like you were doing quite well, so why stop?" Due to my curiosity, I had let down my guard and found myself answering, explaining that I hated how regimented it was. The oddest part was that sometimes my responses surprised me. I was completely truthful about everything from my relationships and how they had ended to why I was out of work and why I liked partying and doing drugs.

It became very clear that Dr. Smith was not like the other doctors and psychologists I had seen. As the questions became very personal, I hesitated. I had promised to cooperate, but I was very aware that my mother was there. As if she sensed my worry, she simply patted me on the leg as if trying to comfort me. I answered all the answers as best I could, attempting to gauge Dr. Smith's reaction to my responses. Unfortunately, Dr. Smith's face never gave anything away. I was good at reading people, so I didn't like the fact that I couldn't glean any information from Dr. Smith.

Pausing, Dr. Smith looked away from me with his calculating eyes and made a few notes on his legal pad before turning to my mother. When he asked my mother about some of my responses, I was astonished and angry as I listened to her disagree with me. When he had asked if I ever felt paranoid, I had answered no, but my mother's answer shocked me. Not only did my mother contradict most of my statements but she went into great detail about my behavior. *Why is she lying?* I wondered. My hands gripped into tight fists as I sat in stunned silence, listening as she told story after story of when my outbursts caused trouble for me, my sister, and my parents. She even told stories of me as a child, when I tried to jump out of our car while we were driving on I-70.

I remembered the stories, but they felt distant and false the way she described them.

Tired of listening, I interrupted. "This is ridiculous." Something in my voice surprised me: doubt. It was as if I wasn't sure if her stories or my memories were accurate.

Dr. Smith leaned back in his seat, taking his glasses off and holding them in his right hand as he looked between me and his notes. Pausing and taking a deep breath before putting his glasses back on, Dr. Smith ignored my interruption and asked me about my explosive reactions, inquiring about why I felt the need to react with such ferocity. Feeling guarded and under attack, I listened to every question carefully before answering. I wasn't going to be caught off guard again. After a bit more than an hour, Dr. Smith finally put down his pen.

Taking off his glasses, he met my eyes, setting his hands down in his lap as he leaned forward. "Kirk, you certainly have ADHD as Dr. Hudson diagnosed in your teens, but there are far more serious problems that we need to address." Dr. Smith picked up my medical file once again, reading the notes of the other psychologists who had worked with me before continuing. "From everything in your file, your tests, your behavior, the notes of the other psychologists, and everything I have heard today, I have no doubt that you have an extremely severe case of bipolar. Although you do exhibit some psychotic symptoms, that is not uncommon with bipolar." I was about to speak but then realized that he wasn't done. "You also have generalized and social anxiety."

"What?" I said, not sure exactly how offended I should be. I didn't feel fear, especially when it came to other people, so how could I have anxiety?

"What exactly does all that mean?" my mother asked, her hand grasping mine as she waited to hear the news. I pulled my hand away, still angry. I had always been fascinated with mental disorders and had taken a few psychology classes that had briefly gone over bipolar, among other mental disorders, so I knew the answer before Dr. Smith began.

"Bipolar has no cure, and it has been shown to get worse with time." My mother was trying her best to hold herself together, but I could tell she was in pain. "The good news is that we have medications that will help your son manage the condition." Dr. Smith paused to give my mother time to think before continuing. "It is my job to be honest so that you, your son, and your family go into his treatment with realistic expectations."

My mother was nervous and held her hands together as she spoke, "I understand. Please continue."

"With such a severe case, even with medication, it is important to realize that there is a strong possibility that he will never lead a normal life." Dr. Smith turned to me as he continued. "I would highly suggest that you also continue to see someone. If you would like to work with someone other than me, I would understand and can give you some names. Bipolar I is a serious disorder and should not be taken lightly. Your son needs treatment, both with medications and weekly sessions, if he hopes to have a chance at maintaining a job or relationship."

I was about to tell Dr. Smith what I thought of him, but my mother spoke first. "I would like to continue seeing you if you have time. Every doctor I spoke with kept bringing up your name, so would you be willing to see us?" I could tell that my mother was clinging to the hope that Dr. Smith would say yes, but as he nodded, she took a deep breath and asked, "I know this is not a polite question, but I must ask. Is there any way that your diagnosis is wrong?"

"Mrs. Miller, you must understand that I do not come to such a devastating diagnosis lightly." Dr. Smith's voice was gentle for the first time as he addressed my mother. "I reviewed your son's file multiple times before today, looking carefully through the many notes and medical information from his doctors and psychologists for anything that might point to something other than bipolar. Unfortunately, everyone your son has seen is highly respected and also believed Kirk was bipolar. Between the results of his psychological tests, the previous psychologists' notes, and everything I have heard today, I am quite comfortable with my assessment. It is my professional opinion that your son needs help."

"I think we should get a second opinion," I said, feeling anger and frustration as I spoke. For the first time in weeks, I felt a hint of energy, but it quickly faded as I sighed and sat back, crossing my arms.

Dr. Smith met my gaze as he spoke. "Kirk, you have every right to seek a second opinion, and I will even give you names, but I must be honest with you. In my opinion, every psychiatrist who reviews this file and speaks with you and your family will come to the same conclusion.

I apologize for breaking such news to you, but this is a serious disorder. Personally, I feel it would be best if you began taking medication immediately. I would also like to see you next week if possible."

My mother did her best to hold back her tears, but a few droplets slid down her cheeks. As for me, I simply stared at Dr. Smith. I hated him and everything about the diagnosis. I didn't have bipolar, and I didn't need medication. Unfortunately, I knew that what I thought was no longer part of the equation. The expert had spoken, and I knew my mother would listen.

Since I was living at home with no job and no money for rent, I had two choices: run away or give the medications and therapy a chance. I wanted to run, and had I been in a manic stage I have no doubt I would've vanished, but I was just coming out of my worst depression. I gave in. As my mother handed Dr. Smith a check she couldn't afford in exchange for a fistful of prescriptions and blood test orders, I had stopped caring. After hearing that there was no cure and I would never be free of medication, I remember clearly wondering if my family would be better off if I was gone.

III. GIVING IN TO MEDICATION

The trip home was long as my mother tried to talk about anything but the heavy truth hanging over us both. I was just looking forward to getting home and taking a long nap that would take me away from reality. I didn't know much about lithium or the other drugs Dr. Smith had written prescriptions for, but I wondered what they did and how they would affect me. I had tried enough drugs that I was slightly curious, but every time I tried to relax, my mind returned to the same moment in the psychiatrist's office. Dr. Smith had been very clear that there was no cure, although we might be able to manage the symptoms and keep my outbursts to a minimum. I didn't care about managing my symptoms, for all I kept hearing was that there was no cure. Knowing that I was going to be on medication for the rest of my life without even a guarantee that I would get better was hard to swallow.

On our way home, my mother stopped by the Walgreens near our house, handing the pharmacist the fistful of prescriptions that needed to be filled along with her credit card. My mother had tried to hide how much the single visit to Dr. Smith had cost, but I had caught a glimpse of the check when she handed it over. Six hundred dollars was far more than my mother or father could afford, and I knew that monthly bills for medication would only add strain to my mother. I didn't feel bad, but I felt angry that my mother had been fooled by a smooth-talking shrink. Years later, I would realize just how correct Dr. Smith had been.

There was only one reason that I would take the medication. I had given my mother my word. When we returned home, I was heading toward the basement door when my mother called out. "Dr. Smith said you should start your medications today."

I sighed and turned back around, walking into the kitchen as my mom carefully read the labels before handing me three pills from the lithium bottle and a tiny round pill from the bottle labeled Klonopin. I didn't hesitate as I tossed the pills into my mouth and stuck my head under the sink. Whatever the pills were, I was confident they wouldn't be nearly as potent as some of the drugs I had taken in the past. I was very wrong. The drugs they gave me to control my swings were stronger than any of the drugs I could get on the street, only these had no positive effects. I must take a brief moment to say that this was how I felt when my mind was lost. The truth is that the current bipolar medications have a part to play in treating bipolar, and I simply can't condemn them as they do save lives.

After swallowing the pills, I turned away from the sink as my mother walked up to me. Her face was drawn and sad as she wrapped her thin arms around my waist. It was clear that Dr. Smith's explanation of what bipolar was had left my mother worried. I had stopped listening when he had explained that I was currently recovering from "a major depressive episode" and that it would take time for the medications to work. What I gathered was that Dr. Smith thought I needed to be carefully monitored. "Are you okay?" my mother asked gently as I pulled away.

"I'm tired," I answered truthfully before turning and vanishing into the basement.

Walking into my basement bedroom that remained dark throughout the day, I collapsed on my bed. The day felt oddly distant and dreamlike. Only now do I realize how odd it was that, on the very day I was diagnosed with a major mental illness, I didn't wonder or worry about my mind or the medications I would be taking for the rest of my life. Had I felt better, I might have smiled at how absurd the psychiatrist had been, but I wasn't ready to smile yet.

Looking over to the clock next to my bed, I saw that it was a bit past four in the afternoon. All I wanted was to escape the world. Figuring I'd watch some television before heading to bed, I didn't give the day much thought. I wondered when I would start feeling energetic again. I know now that what I was craving was to feel manic again, but at the time I simply thought I was tired of feeling worthless. Even before the medications had a chance to begin to work, my depression continued to fade. For the first day in weeks I went twenty-four hours without thinking of suicide. Since I had just begun the medication, I was torn between wondering if it was working or if I was simply feeling better.

The truth is that the medications don't work that fast, and Dr. Smith had been correct that I was recovering from a deep depression. I didn't really give it much thought; I was just glad to feel the darkness lifting. My so-called "swings" were as natural to me as breathing, making it impossible to look inward and see the truth of my situation. Only now can I look back and objectively analyze what I was going through. After watching some television, I returned to my room and collapsed on my bed. When I closed my eyes, sleep came hard and fast.

The next morning, I awoke to a gentle knock at my door. "Kirk, can Mom and I come in?" my sister asked.

"Come on in," I answered slowly as I rubbed my eyes. I didn't feel any different from taking the doctor's medication, but I hadn't expected to. There was a sense of slight satisfaction that the medication hadn't done anything, but that satisfaction vanished as my mother and sister came in with concern on their faces. "What's wrong?"

My sister came over and gave me a big hug. "Mom and Dad told me everything. How are you holding up?"

I shook my sister off, annoyed at being reminded of the previous day. Until my sister had brought it up, the previous day's events were absent from my thoughts. "I'm fine."

My mom extended her hand, and I stared at it. "Your father said that you could take your pills in the morning or at night." My dad was a great pharmacist and would have made an amazing doctor. I didn't listen to many people, but when it came to medicine, I listened when my dad gave advice. "I also wanted to remind you that next week we have an appointment with Dr. Smith again. Your father would like to come as well, if that's okay."

It was clear that everyone was worried, and I wasn't in the mood to deal with anyone. Taking the pills out of my mother's hand and throwing them into my mouth, I reached for the bottle of water that I kept next to my bed, swallowing the pills before speaking harshly. "I'll take the damn pills in the morning, but I could use a day without being interrogated." My family, friends, and loved ones never deserved to be spoken to in the way I often did. They cared for me and often took the brunt of my frustration, anger, or sadness at the world I saw. Although I'm a completely different person now, it pains me to look at how I treated those who cared for me and see the trauma I caused everyone who grew close to me. "I hope what happened yesterday will remain within the family." I wasn't crazy and certainly didn't want any women I dated or my friends to think otherwise. It was the first time I felt the stigma that was forever intertwined with my life.

"Of course we won't tell anyone," my mother and sister said at nearly the same time.

"Just leave me alone, okay?" I said coldly.

Instead of asking why I wanted to be alone or trying to make me feel better, my mother and sister just nodded and left the room. The fact that my mother and sister did not like leaving things unresolved only made the ease of getting them to leave feel odd. My sister was always trying to lift my spirits or calm me down in an effort to keep the family from fighting. It was a burden she should not have tried to shoulder, but I'm not sure our family would have survived without her. My father was always the calm one in our family, but my mother fed off of my energy, making every swing I went through affect the entire family. Many times, my explosions caused fights between my mother and father, again leaving my sister struggling to calm everyone down. I do admit that our family put on a good show. To everyone who didn't live with us, we looked like a normal family. The truth, however, was that I was putting a strain on everyone close to me, and we were far from normal. Our family was suffering, and I have no illusions that I was not responsible for a large part of it.

After my door closed, I heard my mother and sister begin to cry. I felt not guilt but annoyance as I covered my ears with my pillows. I was agitated, but I didn't feel any more energetic than the previous day. As I rolled onto my side, my stomach rumbled. It had been a while since I had eaten, and I was hungry, but I still wasn't ready to leave my room. Well aware that my sister and mother had probably spent hours researching bipolar, I wasn't in the mood to talk about my supposed insanity. Many might claim that I was in denial, but the terrifying part of bipolar is that even at the peaks of my mania or depression, I couldn't see the reality of my actions or life. Even with the medications, I never felt like there was anything wrong with me.

Closing my eyes, I just wanted to sleep. For the next few days, I came out of my room only for food and to take the medications that were supposed to help me to be "normal." It was always hard to tell how long I would stay in the late stage of my depression, but after a few days I began to feel a bit better. I certainly wasn't feeling great, but I shaved, showered, and ate. My depression was fading, but following closely behind it was another round of mania. It was always just a matter of time.

Looking back, perhaps the clearest sign that my depression was fading was that colors seemed brighter, unlike the darker shades of gray I would see when I was in the final stage of my depression. My favorite color when I was growing up was always black, not because I liked black but because I truly didn't like any color. With the aid of hindsight, my darkest depressions always seemed to dim the world around me into pale shades. That dimming was usually the first sign that I was heading to a deeper depression.

After the diagnosis, nothing really changed. My family continued to walk on eggshells around me, although I didn't know it at the time. Wondering if the medication was actually working, I spoke with my dad. He had a knack for explaining medications in a way that always answered my questions. That morning, my dad and I were sitting alone, giving me the opportunity to ask him some questions while my sister and mother were away. "So, what is lithium?"

"It is a medication prescribed in order to stabilize your moods. It controls the flow of sodium through your muscle and nerve cells," my dad answered gently. "It's a potent drug, but if monitored, it can be very useful."

"So how does it work?"

"No one really knows," my dad answered honestly as he stood up from the kitchen table and looked at my prescription. "You're just starting, so it will take a few weeks to get your blood level stabilized."

"So that's why I have to take a blood test every week?" My father nodded and walked back to the table.

"Correct. They have to be careful with such a potent medication, so Dr. Smith is doing a good job. Usually it's used in combination with other medication, but I'm guessing that Dr. Smith may want to get your lithium level stable before adding anything else."

I couldn't get past what he had said earlier in the conversation, asking, "They really don't know how it works?"

My father nodded. "Many of the drugs they use to treat bipolar are new. Because we don't know what causes bipolar, we really don't know how many of the bipolar medications help, even if we know how they affect the body. They do work, so you need to listen to Dr. Smith and take your meds. Just because no one really understands how the drugs work doesn't mean that they haven't been shown to be effective."

"So—" I hesitated and then decided to finish my question. "Do you think I'm bipolar?"

My dad paused, scratching his thick brown beard as he sighed. "I'm afraid if I look at your behavior as objectively as I can …" my father paused, his bushy eyebrows lowering over his eyes as he looked down. "I would say that it makes some sense."

"Even you think I'm nuts?" I said angrily as I picked up my bowl of cereal and stood up. Walking over to the sink, I dropped my bowl of cereal into the sink, ignoring the noise it made.

"Kirk, you know that I don't think you're crazy, but perhaps the medications will help," my father said gently, always the optimist. I shook my head and walked away.

Over the next month, I took multiple blood tests and saw Dr. Smith twice more. My lithium dosage was increased dramatically, and I was prescribed three more medications to help keep my bipolar in check. To say that the medications did affect me is a gross understatement, but they didn't stop the swings. The medications may have helped slow how often I had a manic or depressive episode, but each mania or depression continued to grow more severe, no matter how much Dr. Smith increased the number or dosage of my medications.

> **Important note:** To everyone reading this memoir, I must make one thing *very* clear. Had I not sought medical help and taken my prescribed medications as directed, I would not be around now to tell my story. As I talk about what happened to me and the side effects I encountered when taking bipolar medications, it is important for everyone dealing with bipolar to fully understand that I strongly support the brilliant researchers and doctors who are currently working on treating bipolar and *do not* condone or advocate any action without the formal advice and guidance of a trained medical professional.

IV.   TRYING TO FIND STABILITY

After a few months of constant blood tests and some setbacks leading to an increase in my medications, I was growing tired of being poked and prodded. Feeling like a lab rat was not working for me, and it felt like my life revolved around medical appointments and sessions with Dr. Smith. With nearly every blood test or session with Dr. Smith, a new medication would be added or my dosage adjusted. Many times, a new drug would be added to counteract the side effects of my current medications. The entire process was tiring, and the only reason that I continued to go was because I had promised my mother. In all respects, even with the medications and sessions with Dr. Smith, I wasn't improving. My swings continued, and the violence of my manic episodes was not lessened, nor were the deep feelings of self-loathing during my depressions. Although only a few months had passed, I had experienced two depressive episodes and one month-long manic episode during which I nearly found myself in jail for fighting.

One of the biggest problems with the frequency of my appointments and medical tests was that it was beginning to cause tension between me and Sara, as I will refer to her. Sara was my girlfriend at the time, and we were quickly becoming involved. Although we were becoming more serious, I wasn't about to tell her about my bipolar. Even if I still felt that nothing was wrong with me, I didn't want others judging me.

I knew that Sara, a soft-spoken girl with striking blue eyes and a kind heart, would not understand. Besides, I didn't feel like I was keeping anything from her as I was still unable to see the reality of my life. As we became more serious, I asked her to move in with me. As always, I was taking actions based on the present, unaware of the complications that living with someone might entail. Since she was already a student at a nearby college, she agreed, and we moved into my parents' basement. She saved some money on rent, and I think my family thought I must be improving if I was able to be stable enough to convince a woman to move in with me. Unfortunately, I was experiencing a long mania, and I was moving too fast with Sara.

When she moved in with me, it became harder to hide what I was going through. I had to schedule all my medical appointments for when she had class and take my medications when she wasn't paying attention. I was actually annoyed with her for inconveniencing me, unaware that I was the one hiding a serious truth from her. As usual, I was unable to see her point of view. Thinking only of myself, I never thought of taking her feelings into account.

After being diagnosed, I was curious to see how other people viewed bipolar. What I found was that the disorder was widely misunderstood and, in many cases, viewed as a mild inconvenience. As I spoke to people about the disorder, keeping it a secret that I had been diagnosed as I asked for their opinions, I found that there were two very distinctive groups. The first group viewed bipolar as an excuse for an individual to act out while avoiding responsibility. These individuals had no sympathy for anyone with bipolar, but not because they were bad people. They simply hadn't dealt with someone with bipolar and had no experience with the devastation the disorder could cause. I couldn't fault them for their lack of understanding, as I was just beginning to research bipolar myself. Although I didn't believe I had bipolar, I was still curious to learn about it. My understanding of what bipolar was came slowly because the only time I was able to research was during the first stage of my mania.

The second group had the opposite view because they had directly seen or been involved with someone with bipolar. These people tightened up even thinking about their experiences and were extremely cautious with their words and opinions. More than once, my gentle questions brought on tears, and many couldn't even talk about their experiences dealing with a loved one who suffered with bipolar. Having seen the true destructive power of bipolar, these individuals spoke of bipolar as if it were a life-threatening disease. To be fair, I agree more with the second group; many whom I spoke to had lost a family member in some tragic way. Each one of these individuals wanted to stay as far away from bipolar as they could. Some told horrific stories of feeling threatened and endangered from just being around their sibling, partner, or husband. With such extreme views, neither group made me feel like making my diagnosis pubic would be a good idea. Therefore, I decided to keep my diagnosis, as false as I felt it to be, a secret from everyone. That included my friends and, of course, Sara.

Keeping it a secret became harder as time went on; the medications began to cause both common and more severe side effects. Not only did I begin to suffer from more common side effects but there were side effects that were not listed, including a complete loss of interest in things like playing the violin or painting. As my side effects began to become severe enough that the people closest to me began to notice, I became quite adept at lying about why I was losing my hair or was having a hard time retaining my short-term memory.

When my lithium dosage was increased to 1,800 milligrams daily, my blood test showed that I was extremely close to a toxic level. Like many people taking large doses of lithium, I developed thyroid problems, and yet another medication was added to a growing list that I was incapable of following. Had my mother not set out my pills, I wouldn't have been able to keep up with all the daily medications I had to take.

As my hair continued to thin, I began to have problems with simple motor skills. My hands would shake so badly that often food would fall from my fork before reaching my mouth. These side effects, along with the mental fog they caused, made me want to stop taking my medications, but I kept my word to my mother and took my pills every morning. Eventually, my mind was so drugged I would stare off into the distance, unable to think or care. As time passed, it seemed that the doctors added a new medication to address each side effect, but the game of balancing my medications became quite frustrating.

Although my family and Dr. Smith thought that I was finally reaching some level of stability, I felt more drugged and sedated than ever, and that included when I was taking drugs like opium and heroin. In many ways, I was surprised how powerful the medications I took really were. My mind, which I had always treasured, felt heavy, and my thoughts were slow and muddled. Luckily, even with the medications, I was still unaware of reality and didn't notice what I had lost or gained.

The worst part was that I wasn't even aware that two of my greatest passions had vanished. Unfinished paintings hung on the walls, and my manuscripts were left incomplete, not that I cared. Everything in my life had become like my manuscripts and paintings: unfinished and unpolished. Although I had appeared to turn a corner, remaining "stable" for nearly two full months, I wasn't happy, nor did I feel like myself. As my medication increased, everything that I had always loved about myself was vanishing. Nearly at the two-month mark, everyone, including me, was in for quite a surprise.

As I was unable to hide my increasingly severe side effects, Sara eventually began to worry, wondering what had happened to the man that she had first fallen for. Just as everyone was beginning to think the medications were working, I fell into a deep depression. Although the time between my swings had been a bit slower, the medications were unable to completely stop those swings or control them once they began. The worst part was that when I did fall into my first depression since starting my treatments, it was far more severe. Since I had seemed stable for two long months, my crash surprised everyone, and Sara had no idea what was happening. As Dr. Smith had warned me on my first visit with him, even with all the medications there was no guarantee that I would, or could, lead a normal life.

This time, as I fell deeper into the pit that was depression, I couldn't stop falling, and my crash was harsher and faster. Unaware of what was happening with me, Sara kept wondering if she had done something to upset me as I rejected her physical advances, even hugs. Unable to communicate with any skill, Sara packed up a travel bag and left to stay with her parents for a few weeks. I did not care that she was gone, and in fact I was lucky she had left when she did, as my depression quickly grew more severe. Feeling hopeless, I wondered why I was even bothering to take my medications as my world lost all color, vibrancy, and joy. My mind was overtaken by the worst darkness I had ever experienced. As I became catatonic, my mother contacted the doctors, who prescribed yet another medication in an attempt to help me. Although I hated Dr. Smith and the other doctors whom I dealt with, I know now that they were trying their best to fight a battle they had no chance of winning.

When Sara returned a month later, my depression had come and gone, only this time, instead of coming to a short-lived neutral state of stability, I felt my mind overtake my medications as the first stage of mania hit me hard. Not only was I spending money I didn't have but also I wasn't sleeping, instead staying up all night writing, painting, or watching television. I was on enough drugs to knock out a horse, but no amount of medication could temper the ferocity of my ups or downs. In fact, as time went on, my swings continued to grow more severe. Even with great help and medications to stabilize and keep me under control, I was losing my mind and my life was being torn apart because of the bipolar that ruled me.

My sudden and intense swings caught my family, my doctor, and Sara by surprise. I was on the maximum allowed dosage of my many medications, so Dr. Smith wasn't sure why I wasn't doing better. He tried his best to stabilize me, but there was nothing he could do. Sara was glad to see me laughing again, but she had never experienced the later stages of my manias, setting her up for quite a rude awakening.

As my mania began to take over, I decided that it was high time I started doing my own research. There had to be something that Dr. Smith could prescribe that wouldn't make my mind feel so dull while helping control the swings that were quickly growing more potent. Although I had lost my passions, I became obsessed with researching bipolar, at least when I was at the beginning stage of my manias.

When Dr. Smith added Depakote, an anticonvulsant medication that had proven to be successful in helping to control bipolar symptoms, my side effects worsened, but my mania continued to build up its strength. Although I continued to crack jokes, when Sara watched my hands shake so badly that I dropped a glass of water, she demanded answers.

"Are you okay? Why do your hands always shake, and how come I feel like you're hiding something from me?"

"I don't know," I lied. "I think the hand tremors run in the family," I responded without a moment's hesitation. I am not proud of it now, but lying had always been an integral part of my life. Reading people and knowing what to say, while also believing the lies I told, was an important part of my self-preservation. Whether it was dealing with a police officer or a girlfriend, lying was like second nature. The most interesting part is that I never really thought about lying; it just came. In retrospect, I was more lost than ever.

"What is going on with you?" Sara asked, tears forming in her eyes. "Last month you wouldn't even hug me, and now you can't stop smiling. Is it something I did, or are you trying to push me away?"

"What?" I snapped, the violence in my voice making Sara's eyes widen. I still didn't believe I had bipolar, and I certainly wasn't going to go around explaining why my hands shook, especially when she couldn't take my word for it. "Why are you attacking me? I already told you, it runs in the family and is no big deal. What is your problem?"

Sara was taken aback, not sure why my eyes were filled with flashes of anger and unfamiliar with me raising my voice. "I didn't mean anything by it. I was just—"

I cut her off. "If you have a problem with me, just say it. Don't dance around the issue." At the time, I had no idea how intimidating or threatening I could be, so when Sara began to cry and pack her travel bags for a second time, I figured we were done. Angry, I raised my voice and spoke sharply. "So, you're going back to your parents?"

Sara just cried, packed a few of her clothes as fast as she could, and ran upstairs and out of the basement. Although Sara had received permission to live at my house, she had not been entirely truthful about our living situation. Her parents held strong religious beliefs and were quite upset when they found out that we were living in the same room. I never knew it was an issue until later that week.

Two days after she left, I received a call from Sara explaining that she would move out unless I proposed. I had scared her, but for some reason, she had forgiven me, and her parents were demanding that we either live apart or move forward. I had never taken ultimatums well, and, without thinking, I hung up the phone and stormed downstairs.

Filled with anger and unable to remember any good things about our relationship, I took her things and threw them into the center of the room. As the phone continued to ring, I ignored it until all of Sara's belongings were packed. When I was done, I finally answered the phone to hear Sara sobbing on the other line.

"I'm sorry I had to tell my parents. I didn't know what to do. I was going to tell you, but you seemed so angry. Can you forgive me and can we move on?" Sara asked with a pleading tone.

Like always, I was reacting to the present, unable to separate reality from my swirling emotions. "No," I said, my voice cold and decisive, "I can't. You made your choice." After all the times Sara had forgiven me, I didn't even consider her feelings or point of view. "Your stuff is packed, and you can pick it up tomorrow." With that I hung up the phone without a second thought. As the phone began to ring again, I leaned down and tore the phone cable out of the jack, tearing the drywall in the process. Again, my broken mind with its twisted realities had ruined another relationship.

Each and every woman I had dated deserved better treatment than I was capable of providing. I wasn't inherently evil or even a bad guy, but my moods and changing views of the world around me made me erratic, irrational, and often mean. Although I was, at times, a good boyfriend, my sharp tongue had not been dulled by the multitude of medications I was taking. Although I was never physically abusive, my explosions always terrified those closest to me.

Although Sara did call a few more times, I never spoke with or saw her again. What impacts me now is the fact that even after ending one of my most serious relationships I didn't feel any regret, pain, or sadness. Later that week, I was given a higher daily dose of lithium and started on another drug called Lamictal. My doctor and family were trying desperately to find something to help stabilize me, but I was still in denial. Not only did I hate taking the medications but the medications also became a scapegoat. For me, the fact that I was still having problems even while taking the medications proved that my problems were the result of the world around me and not due to any mental disorder.

Two weeks after I broke up with Sara and started yet another medication, my swings continued to grow more severe. There were very brief moments when my family saw a flash of the real person I was and the potential I had, but those fleeting moments only brought my family a false sense of hope that always left them disappointed.

Although my breakup should've affected me to some degree, my mania was gaining traction. As it entered the second stage, I found my way back down to Denver and its many bars and clubs. The risks I took with casual romantic encounters and illicit drugs were more perilous and daring than ever before. Taking 1,800 milligrams of lithium, 450 milligrams of Lamortigine, and four milligrams of Clonazepam per day should've made it hard for me to even get out of bed, but my mania was stronger than ever.

On that Friday I was at one of my favorite clubs drinking when I saw one of my best friends. I had known Ming since the sixth grade, and we had always been very close. Since he still lived in the mountains where we had both grown up, I was surprised to run into him and was glad to see him. Unlike me, he didn't drink or do drugs, nor had he ever done so. The only reason he ever came to clubs was to relax, socialize, and blow off some of the stress that came with running his family's restaurant.

Since I had gotten to the club early, I had been able to secure a small table. Seeing Ming, I called his name, laughing at the look on his face when he saw me. Since most of my close friends had no idea of how I spent my manic weekends, his surprise was understandable.

"Ming," I shouted, "get over here!"

Born in Hong Kong, Ming was an impressive guy, speaking three languages while managing two of his family's restaurants. He was always well-dressed and mature. Ming's thin frame moved easily through the crowd as he walked over to the table and sat down. "I wasn't expecting to see you here," he said, adding, "It's good to see you."

Always one of my best friends, Ming was perhaps the most honorable and stand-up guy I knew. As always, he was overdressed for the club, wearing slacks, polished black shoes, and a stylish tan jacket that looked expensive. I had always liked that Ming knew who he was and didn't care what others thought.

"It's been too long," I responded before asking, "What are you doing down in Denver without calling me?"

"I tried giving you a call, but you never pick up," Ming answered truthfully. He wasn't wrong. "I wanted to let you know that we sold the restaurants and I'm going to be applying to the University of Colorado."

Pleased that Ming was moving on with his own life, I smiled. "That's great, bro. It's about time you did something for yourself." Ming had not been happy with his situation, and I was glad to see that he was moving forward with his life. "Let me buy you a drink in celebration."

"Thanks, Kirk, but I'm okay. Just here to dance and have some fun." Although I went to clubs to drink and flirt, Ming had always amazed me with his ability to have fun without the aid of alcohol, drugs, or an agenda. He was one of the more secure men I knew.

"So when are you moving down here?"

Ming shrugged his shoulders. "I'm actually trying to figure that out. I need to find a place to rent."

"What?" I leaned forward, meeting his gaze as I shook my head. "There is no way you're renting when we have plenty of room at my house. Can you handle sleeping on a futon?" The idea of having one of my best friends as a roommate sounded perfect to me.

"What about you and Sara?" Ming asked. "I thought she was living with you."

"That's over," I said casually.

"You broke up?" Ming looked surprised, not only at the news but also at how relaxed I seemed. "What happened? The last I heard was that you two were getting serious."

I shrugged my shoulders. "Some things just end."

"All of your relationships end," Ming said, trying to smile but unable to hide his concern. "Are you okay?"

Lifting a shot of tequila into the air, I laughed and nodded. "Same shit, different day." Although Ming never really cursed, my words were a phrase he and I had used many times, making both of us laugh. Downing the shot before chasing it with a lemon, I added, "Seriously, bro, I'm good. It was never going to work. She actually tried to trick me into proposing." Although this was not how things had happened, it was the way I remembered the events that led to the relationship's sudden end.

"Well, for what it's worth, I'm sorry."

"You're a good guy, Ming," I said before asking, "So you think you can live with me as a roommate?"

"Probably not," Ming said jokingly as he laughed. "If it's okay with your family, that would be great. Certainly better than some of the apartments I was looking at."

Knowing that my entire family viewed Ming more as my brother than as a friend, I already knew they would love to have him stay with us. "You're family, bro," I said as I waved down the waitress to order another shot. "Seriously, we'd love to have you."

Ming nodded. "Well, then I'll give your parents a call so we can work out the details."

"Now I have a reason to celebrate," I said as the waitress set down another shot. I drank it quickly before looking at my friend, saying, "We're going to have a blast."

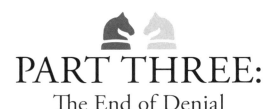

PART THREE:
The End of Denial

:: Desperate Times and Desperate Measures ::

I.   BIPOLAR UNMASKED

When our family first discussed Ming moving in, my parents were very hesitant. They loved Ming and were not worried about him, but they were concerned about me ruining a valued friendship due to my disorder. Although they felt I should tell Ming the truth, I refused, not wanting anyone to know, especially one of my best friends. Eventually I was able to convince my family that having him there might help keep me stable. Two weeks later Ming moved in.

When Ming moved into the basement my mania was still in charge. As my mania began to increase in intensity, I went out nearly every night—drinking, socializing, and using continually harder drugs as I continued to slip further from reality. Since I only socialized with my friends when in a manic stage, Ming didn't think my behavior was any different from what he had seen before. Although he never used drugs and didn't really like drinking, he was aware of some of my activities and never judged me. Quickly finding a job that kept him busy, he avoided seeing my more radical and life-threatening choices.

To me, the risks I took, whether drugs, one-night stands, or fights were not risks at all but were simply part of my warped reality. I was at my most charming and likable during my early manic stages, attracting good girls and friends, but as my mania grew more intense, everything was intensified. Near the end of the month I stumbled into the kitchen after a long night of drinking and socializing. The sun was up, and just as I took my pills, Ming walked into the kitchen. I hadn't noticed him as I took my handful of medications, drinking water to push the pills down. Feeling eyes on me, I turned to see Ming and felt my eyes widen. Ming looked concerned as he pointed to the handful of pills I still needed to take.

"Are you sick, Kirk?" Ming asked, his eyes moving from my handful of pills to my eyes. "Why are you taking all those pills?"

"It's medication for my ADD," I lied, surprised at how quickly I had come up with a perfect explanation. Due to all of the precarious situations I always found myself in, my ability to lie had become imperative to my survival, especially as my activities and the individuals I was around grew more dangerous. The only problem with lying was that it had become more comfortable than telling the truth. Worse was the fact that I could actually believe the lies I told. Although I was taking my medications every day, my mind was still slipping further away from what most people would consider normal, not that I cared.

Unfortunately, my father had just refilled my ADD medication, and it was sitting on the counter next to Ming. As smart as he was, he looked at my hand and then at the prescription before gently prying. "That's a ton of pills," Ming added, knowing that I was aware he had caught my lie, but he didn't press it as he sat down at the kitchen table, speaking as if nothing were different. "I just got a call from Albert. He wants to go out to celebrate his birthday."

Relieved that the issue had vanished, I finished taking my medication before speaking. "Really? It's been a while since I've seen Albert."

"It's been a long time for me too. Albert was wondering if you and I wanted to meet him at Market." Market was one of my favorite clubs down in Denver with great music, a large dance floor, and a large bar with easy access to alcohol. Had I understood my moods, I would never have exposed Ming to my manic side, but I was just excited to hang out with Ming and Albert.

"I'm in," I quickly said, excited to hang out with Ming because

I had hardly seen him lately between his work schedule and my late hours out.

"He was thinking Friday night," Ming responded before taking a sip of his orange juice. "I thought we should invite your sister, just so she can get out and relax."

My sister had just had a bad breakup with a boyfriend who had never been right for her, and Ming was right: she did need some relaxation. After growing up around my constant chaos, Chandi tended to date men who were nearly as damaged as I. Thinking Ming had a good point, I nodded. "I bet she'd love to come. Let me confirm with her, but you can tell Albert that we'll see him there."

Friday came and Ming was happy to be the designated driver. Aware that I partied quite often, my sister had never been out with me and had no idea of the risk she and Ming were taking by going out with me in my current state. I still believe the only reason she had agreed to come was to watch over me. Everyone in my family could sense that I was in a manic state. The only one who wasn't aware was Ming.

With the three of us in Ming's nice car, we headed down to Denver as I kept my sister and Ming laughing with a barrage of jokes. Had I been more aware, I would've noticed that my sister was watching me as she always had, wanting to help and protect me, unaware that it was she that needed protection.

When we arrived at the club, Albert was waiting for us. After paying to get in, Ming and my sister were wishing Albert a happy birthday while I walked straight for the bar. The long, oval bar was at the center of the club with three to six bartenders working at any given time. Since we had arrived early, I was able to walk right up and make an order without waiting.

"Four shots of tequila, please." I figured two drinks for me and two to start off Albert's birthday seemed reasonable.

"Do you want to start a tab, hun?" The thin bartender was dressed in a sexy shirt, her blonde hair curled and pulled back. She quickly poured the shots with ease.

"I'd love to," I said as I reached for my credit card and a few dollars for a tip. "Thanks."

The blonde bartender smiled and gave me a wink before moving on to the next customer. Drinking the first shot, I felt a wave of energy hit me as I turned, waving Albert over. As the same bartender came by, I caught her. "Would you please pour another?"

She nodded and quickly poured the shot with a quick flick of her wrist. "I'll keep them coming if you want."

"Sounds like a plan," I said as Albert walked up. Turning my attention to Albert, I picked up one shot for him and another for me. Handing Albert his shot, I held up the glass before saying, "Here's to having a wild birthday."

Albert was a great guy, and although he wasn't into drugs, he did drink. That was nice as both my sister and Ming did not. I had been out drinking with strangers the last few nights, so it was fun to have a good friend to share some drinks with.

"Cheers," Albert said as we both drank our shots, Albert coughing from the sting of the tequila. Knowing that my sister and Ming wouldn't be up for an all-night outing, I figured there was no reason to pace myself as I picked up and drank my third shot. I wasn't really supposed to drink or do drugs, as the psychiatrist had explained that doing so could affect my medications. Normally I wouldn't have even thought about my psychiatrist, but I was with my sister and figured she would object to multiple shots. I wouldn't have hidden my drinking, but I wasn't in the mood to be hassled.

Albert was still chasing his drink with a lemon when he noticed I was holding a second shot for him. Laughing, he took the shot and said, "So you weren't kidding about the wild birthday, were you?"

"I never kid about fun." Pausing, I slowly scanned the club before looking back to Albert. "Should we get a table?" There weren't many tables as it was more of a dance club, but since we had arrived early, there were a few open.

"If you want," Albert said as I hoped my third shot would kick in shortly.

The strange thing about my mania was that the faster my mind was moving, the slower everything else felt. People around me seemed to be moving in slow motion. The music pumping through the speakers felt good as the vibrations shook the floor. I was completely unaware that I felt any different than earlier that day, but my mania had drastically intensified, making me crave more alcohol or drugs. I was later told that

I was trying to self-medicate as the medications I was taking weren't strong enough to slow my racing mind.

There was nothing different about that particular night, but my view of the present moment was always a reflection of my current mental state. Had I had a terrible experience the previous night, I wouldn't have remembered; my focus was always on the moment. This was especially true during my manic episodes, when everything was centered around fun, socializing, alcohol, and drugs.

Because I never looked back or forward, I never felt regret or fear. This was not helpful in helping me make proper decisions. It was almost as if the bipolar were protecting me from seeing the devastation I always left in my wake or the bridges I had burned. I now know that this strange inability to see beyond my current mood was not unique to me. In fact, nearly every bipolar individual I ever met or interacted with expressed the same sensation of being a slave to their instant swings, unable to grasp the impact of their decisions or look back with a clear mind to learn from past mistakes. Had I not been intoxicated by my mania, I would have known that three shots of tequila were more than enough for starting the night out.

When the bartender handed me two more shots, I downed both and ordered a Long Island for myself. "Should you be drinking that much?"

I turned, realizing my sister was standing there. "I came out to relax. Can you cut me some slack?"

My sister was not happy with my drinking, but she could sense that I was on the edge. "Just take it slow," she said carefully before walking away, probably trying to avoid watching me. Had I been aware of anything but the restlessness I felt, I would've noticed the worried look on her face. I was no fool and knew that alcohol and drugs were never good for me, yet the drive for them was always intense when I was manic. I still have no idea how I avoided addiction. Perhaps my inability to function when depressed kept me from forming steady habits.

After my sister walked away, Albert set down his empty shot glass and smiled. Unlike Ming, Albert was a big guy. Although he was short, he was stocky and had plenty of muscle. He and I had spent more than a few nights drinking together, so he wasn't surprised to see me drinking so heavily. "It's great to see you, man. I really appreciate you and Ming helping me celebrate in style."

"It's the least we could do," I responded while Albert scanned the quickly thickening crowd in order to find Ming and my sister.

"Shall we go sit with Ming and your sister?"

I could barely hear Albert as the music of the club pounded loudly, the bass hitting my body and making it difficult to hear him. Once I realized what he had asked, I shook my head. I wasn't in the mood to have my sister monitor me. "No, but you go for it."

I stood for a moment, watching Albert walk toward my sister and Ming. The harder I tried to calm my mind, the more it seemed to race out of control. My ability to focus was now nonexistent. Worse still was the restlessness that I felt. Eventually my need to move and use up the energy I felt flowing through me became overwhelming.

Walking through the quickly growing crowd and onto the dance floor, a guy bumped into me as I held my Long Island iced tea. Typically, I would've said something, but all I wanted to do was move. Usually I didn't like to dance, but at the moment I was drawn to any activity that would either keep me distracted from my own thoughts or help burn what felt like an eternal spring of energy.

The pulse of the music was enjoyable as I danced, each beat striking my body, daring me to stop. Although I wanted to move faster, I didn't want to spill my drink. As more people moved onto the dance floor, I decided to look for a place to set down my glass. Seeing a table of three girls looking at me and giggling, I walked over. All three women were pretty, but there was one girl wearing a silky gray dress who caught my attention. She had curly black hair that fell down her cheeks, framing her heart-shaped face and dark hazel eyes. Seeing that I was walking in their direction, the three girls blushed, acting as if they hadn't noticed me. I figured they had just noticed how bad a dancer I was, but that didn't bother me.

Like most times when my mania was threatening to peak, I was bold and fearless. My mania had always made approaching women easier for me, but only when it was growing out of control. When I arrived at the table, I gave a gentle smile, leaned in so that the girls could hear me, and asked, "Can I buy you ladies a drink?" The girls nodded, so I smiled and reached out my hand to introduce myself. "I'm Kirk. It's nice to meet you all." Extending my hand to the girl in the gray dress first, I asked, "Was my dancing really bad, or do I have hope?"

All three girls laughed, instantly relieving any tension they might have felt. The black-haired woman reached out and shook my hand. "My name is Lilly, and no, your dancing wasn't bad." Lilly's dark brown eyes were kind as she pointed to a chair. "You can sit down if you want."

I didn't want to sit, but I wanted another drink, and Lilly had caught my attention, so I pulled up a barstool and joined them. After ordering all the girls a drink and enjoying a few laughs, I looked at Lilly and stood up, offering my hand. "I'm still in the mood to dance if you are up to it." I was usually not such a forward guy, but aside from all the bad that came with mania, confidence and lack of fear were two perks that I did enjoy.

As Lilly took my hand, I nodded to her friends before leading her onto the dance floor. The restlessness I felt had not faded, but being out on the dance floor helped, as did having someone to dance with. As the music pulsed through the dance floor, Lilly put her arms around my neck and pulled me closer. All the alcohol I had downed that night should've been kicking in, but my mania was stronger. I certainly wasn't feeling any more relaxed; however, I was enjoying my time with Lilly. Although I was having a hard time focusing, Lilly and I were hitting it off.

"How about we take a break?" Lilly asked when the song we were dancing to ended. When I nodded, she took my hand and led me off the dance floor. I was expecting to head back toward her friends, but Lilly led me to a different table and sat down. "I'm up for another cocktail if you are."

I sat down and smiled. "Sure thing. What do you want?"

It was then that Lilly leaned forward and kissed me, surprising me with how forward she was. After the long and gentle kiss, she moved her lips next to my ear and whispered, "My place isn't far away, and I've had a rough week. Would you like to ditch this place and have a cocktail where we can talk?"

I had always taken foolish chances when it came to matters of the fairer sex, and I was about to say yes when Albert came over. The alcohol that still wasn't silencing my thoughts had hit my friend hard as he leaned on the table, nearly slipping off as he tried to stay on his feet. Puffing out his chest, Albert leaned toward Lilly and said, "Aren't you a beautiful little lady?"

Although Albert was a good guy, I could tell that his swaying and slurred speech were bothering Lilly. Acting fast, I introduced them to each other. "Albert, this is Lilly. Lilly, this is my good friend Albert, who's celebrating his birthday tonight—and doing a good job, from what I can tell."

Lilly let down her guard, nodding to Albert and giving him a polite smile. Behind her smile, I could tell she was not pleased that we had been interrupted. "Happy birthday, Albert. If you don't mind, I—"

Before Lilly could finish, Albert sat down between us. Slightly annoyed, Lilly stood up and straightened her short gray dress before walking to my side. Leaning forward to reach the Cosmopolitan I had ordered for her, she kissed my cheek and said, "When you're ready to go, just come and get me." With that, she kissed me once more and walked away as Albert stared at me.

"You dog!" Albert said, playfully hitting my shoulder. "I still say she'd be kissing me if I had seen her first."

I just laughed, not willing to pass up such an invitation. I was about ready to go and tell Ming I didn't need a ride home when my mania again grew in intensity. Suddenly, my restlessness turned into a light paranoia. There were a group of guys standing behind Albert, and although I know now that they were simply hanging out, at the time I felt like they were watching me. I hadn't even noticed Albert was still talking when I stood up, glaring at one of the guys who had looked my way. Lifting up my hands, I shouted, my words faint against the booming music that was making my ears ring. "You have a problem with me?"

The guy I was addressing tried his best to ignore me, but that wasn't going to work. "What's wrong, bro?" Albert asked as I stood there staring.

"I'm just sick of that guy glaring at me."

"What are you talking about, bro? Just relax."

I couldn't relax. I felt like the guy had a problem with me, and I had an overwhelming sense that I might need to protect myself. Usually, I could have blamed this aggressive behavior on alcohol, but these same feelings had happened multiple times when I was completely sober. The impulse to fight made me dangerous because neither I nor anyone else was able to predict how I would react. Lacking the ability to see my situation clearly, I was unable to recognize that the guy I was threatening was not alone.

The anger I felt was hot, and the fact that I felt more and more eyes turning toward me and judging me certainly didn't help. Feeling indestructible, I was ready for a confrontation, but just as I was walking past Albert to confront the guy I was looking at, Albert caught my arm and held me back. "Dude, it's my birthday. Settle down. Besides, he's got at least six friends. It's not that I wouldn't back you up, but I'm a bit drunk."

I was breathing heavily and even Albert seemed hesitant to hold me back, but as the guys at the next table began to stand up in preparation for a confrontation, my sister and Ming walked over. Although Ming and my sister had no idea that I was near blowing a gasket, my sister leaned forward. "I need to leave soon. Is that okay with you?"

The tone of my sister's voice was so gentle that most of the anger I was feeling faded for the moment. Fortunately, I had not hit my peak yet. Once I was fully manic and had a goal in mind, there was nothing that could calm me or keep me from acting.

"Do you mind if I dance a bit longer?" I asked, and my sister nodded.

"Not at all. Ming and I will be waiting at the front. Is thirty minutes enough?"

I wanted to say no, but I needed to catch up with Lilly before I knew what I would do. I nodded. Despite the alcohol I had consumed, I still didn't feel drunk. I was beginning to feel relaxed, but that didn't mean that I was in control. "Okay," I said, heading off into the crowd.

By the second time my sister found me after I lost track of time, her tone had changed, and I could tell she was upset. "It's been nearly forty-five minutes."

"I'm sorry. I have to catch up with someone and might not need a ride home. Can you give me fifteen more minutes?"

As always, I was being selfish, but my sister nodded. "Come tell us as soon as you know, okay?"

"Deal," I said, not wasting time as I moved into the crowd looking to find Lilly before leaving. I hadn't seen her in a while and was wondering if she had left, but finally I found her sitting and laughing with her friends near the back of the club. When Lilly saw me, she smiled and stood up to greet me. I wanted to stay, but I had promised my sister and knew that Ming was also waiting for me. "So, Kirk, I thought you had vanished without saying good-bye."

"I want to stay, but everyone is bugging me to leave. I wouldn't go, but my sister is here and it's my friend's birthday. Can I give you a call sometime?"

Lilly took a pen out of her small wrist purse and leaned away and over the table, writing her number on a napkin before standing back up and handing it to me. "Call me tomorrow, okay?" As I reached for the napkin, she pulled it just out of my reach and put one hand on my chest, meeting my eyes with hers. "I like you, so don't play any games."

"Tomorrow," I said as she handed me the number. I leaned in and gave her a quick kiss on the cheek before turning away and moving toward the club's exit. Although I had enough energy to dance until dawn, I figured the night had been successful. Also, once we dropped off my sister, there were also good clubs in Boulder if Ming was okay driving.

I met up with my sister and Ming, and we all wished Albert a happy birthday. Ming made sure that Albert had a safe ride home before we left the club and parted ways. The conversation during our walk back to the car felt one-sided as I teased my sister for needing to be up early. I wasn't aware that both Ming and Chandi were upset with me.

When we got into the car and began our trip home, my hope of enjoying the rest of the evening was quickly shattered as my sister scolded me. "You knew I had to be up early, and it is three hours later than you promised we would leave."

I snapped, lashing out with a violent tone and harsh language. "You didn't even have to come. Ming and I only invited you out of pity." As always, I had a way of honing in on someone's insecurities or pain so that my verbal attacks would be more effective.

Ming jumped in, his voice calm as he talked to my sister. "That isn't true, Chandi. Kirk, you owe your sister an apology."

"You two are ganging up on me!" I shouted as my mania skipped from the second stage to a peak. My sister and my best friend suddenly felt like distant enemies who had me cornered in a car. Taken over by roaring emotions and fed by a thick river of energy, I launched into a tirade of curse words that brought my sister to tears and caused Ming to yell.

"Calm down, damn it!" Ming shouted as I began hitting his dashboard as hard as I could, but there was no chance that anyone could reason with me. When I began to try to unlock the door and open it while we were driving on the highway, my sister began to panic.

I didn't hear what she said, but Ming continued to relock the doors and attempt to drive as I hit the windows, cursed, and threatened both Ming and my sister. For me, the twenty-minute drive felt like an eternity. I just wanted to get out of the car, even if that meant breaking down the door. "Let me out!"

"Fine," Ming said with disgust, slowing the car and beginning to pull over.

"Please don't pull over, Ming." My sister pleaded as I continued to try and get out of the car. My curse words were flying so fast that they weren't understandable. At that moment, clawing at the door and shouting, I was more animal than man.

Finally arriving home, I got out of the car and charged into the house, slamming every door I passed and cursing loudly enough to wake my parents and gain our neighbors' attention. When my parents rushed down to see what was wrong, I had already grabbed the portable phone and gone into the basement and out the back door. Our house backed to open space, so I quickly jumped the back fence and kept dialing Mike. I didn't know where I was going, but I knew I had to flee.

That night's outburst had been the most violent and aggressive that I had ever had, and I was on multiple medications that were supposed to help keep me from such explosions. I'm sure that alcohol played a part in the outburst, but the sad truth was that even when I was sober, my explosions were getting more severe.

I walked for hours as my family desperately looked for me and called the police. I was paranoid enough to avoid any cars that were out driving, which is probably the only reason I avoided being arrested that night. I was wild and angry, and I have no doubt that I would have attacked anyone who came near me—cop, friend, or foe.

After a few hours of walking, my mania vanished, and once again I was plunged into a deep and heavy depression. For me and many others with bipolar, the change from depression to mania is a slow process, but that is not the case when swinging the other way, at least for me. Suddenly tired and unable to think, I found my way back home. I snuck into the house and climbed into my bed.

Amazingly enough, the next morning, Ming came into my room. "Listen, Kirk, I'm really sorry about how everything went down last night." Although my depression was holding strong, it was still in the beginning stages, so I was able to function. The truth was that I remembered my own version of the previous night. I hadn't had enough to drink to affect my memory, but my view on what happened was tainted by my oncoming depression.

I spoke quietly as I was in no mood for talking. "No problem, bro. I'm sorry too. Let me get some sleep and we'll talk later." In hindsight, there was no reason Ming should've been the one to apologize.

After the wild night, my family felt obligated to explain to Ming that I had been diagnosed with bipolar and that I hadn't been myself the previous night. As I would've expected from Ming, he never treated me differently. He did, however, move out a few months later for his own personal reasons. After that night, Ming's eyes were open to what bipolar really was. He admitted that before seeing it with his own eyes, he had always thought of bipolar as a simple and harmless disorder. I lost many friends because of bipolar, but luckily Ming is still one of my closest friends. I never did call Lilly.

II.   THE BEST GIFT BIPOLAR EVER GAVE ME

During that summer, I had a total of three major episodes, two manic and one depressive. The outburst that rocked my friendship with Ming sent me into a deep depression that lasted nearly a month. During that time, Dr. Smith tried his best to adjust my medication and try different combinations, but everyone was beginning to believe that I would never be able to live a normal life. I was, as I had always been, oblivious to my own situation. As the summer was coming to a close and I was coming out of one of my longest and darkest depressions, I stumbled across one of my old crushes from high school.

Nicoal was a beautiful Korean woman whom I had liked back in high school. Our age difference had made it impossible for us to date at the time, but knowing she had graduated and was now eighteen changed our situations. I asked her if she would be interested in going out to dinner and was pleased when she said yes. I planned a nice date for the two of us to get reacquainted.

The dinner was great. I took her to a small restaurant up in the mountains. Talking with her was easy, relaxing, and we hit it off. Not sure if she even realized that I viewed the dinner as an official date, I tried to read her, but she gave no hints as to her interest in me. Unlike her, I had dated quite a bit, but Nicoal was a new experience. The connection we had was powerful and more than physical.

After an enjoyable meal, it was time for her to go home, so we walked to the parking lot and stopped beside her car. Knowing it would be the last time I saw her before she left for college, I wanted to make my feelings perfectly clear. As the first stage of mania made me bold and daring, I took a chance. Reaching out and pulling her close, I kissed her. At first, she melted into my arms, but then she stiffened up and pulled away, looking flustered. The kiss had been amazing, but something was wrong. Nicoal quickly said good-bye and got into her car.

The next day she called me. "We need to talk," she said, her voice sounding angry, which I wasn't expecting.

"Okay," I responded slowly. "What do we need to talk about?"

"You were completely out of line last night."

"What?"

Nicoal sounded flustered as she explained herself. "You didn't even ask if I was dating someone, yet you had the audacity to kiss me. Why would you—"

I cut Nicoal off before she could continue. "I am so sorry. I had no idea you were seeing anyone, and I didn't want to pass up the chance to show you how I felt," I answered honestly.

"Although I'm leaving for college, my boyfriend and I had not decided whether to end things or not. I should've told you my situation, but I didn't realize you were interested in me, and the kiss just caught me off guard." There was a long pause before Nicoal added, "I'm not saying that I didn't enjoy it …"

Nicoal was younger than I, and I knew she had only dated one person, making me realize that my actions had probably been surprising and new to her. Not wanting to lose my chance with her, I quickly added, "You have every right to be mad at me, but I had a great time and wouldn't have done that if I had known your situation." As I spoke, I was fairly certain that I would've kissed her regardless of her situation. There was a heat between us that I couldn't explain, and it was intoxicating.

Hearing a sigh on the other end of the line, I just waited until Nicoal spoke. "I had a great time, but I leave in a few days. Perhaps we can catch up next summer."

Yeah right, I thought at first, figuring she would head off to college and find someone there. Although I didn't believe the words, I said, "Until next summer."

"You could always e-mail me," Nicoal added, surprising me.

Nicoal was young, but she had a great mind and a glowing personality, and she was beautiful. Figuring there was no reason to shut the door while it was open, I responded honestly. "I will."

To my surprise, we did stay in touch. There were lapses when I was depressed and never checked my e-mail, but overall, we talked once every week or so. Since we weren't exclusive, I continued to go out when my mania took over. Having no idea if she was even going to come back, I would occasionally find myself enjoying short romances. What was odd was that I would often think of Nicoal after ending a relationship. Even my serious relationships had never held my attention the way Nicoal did. I wasn't sure if it was the idea of Nicoal or that we had a true spark.

Although my romantic endeavors didn't seem to change, my willingness to try more intense and serious drugs had changed. My manias had become so out of control that I often thought my head would explode. This feeling made me seek out stronger drugs, and eventually I found a few that were hard enough to quiet my mind for a few hours. What little money I made from playing at weddings or social events quickly vanished, spent on drugs powerful enough to provide me a few hours of respite from my own mind. As I said before, I have no doubt that only my depressions and my inability to function during my deepest downs saved me from becoming addicted or overdosing. In short, it was my darkest times that kept me alive.

As the year went on I continued to deteriorate, but I tried my best to e-mail Nicoal when I was functioning. I had been treating my bipolar for over a year with powerful medications, but things continued to get worse. Although I didn't see it, I heard this whenever my mother or sister came to a therapy session with me. Not once did I agree, as I saw my reality through eyes controlled by a twisted mind.

For many people suffering with bipolar, the medications do take away their intoxicating highs or make them feel sluggish and even sick. I was no different, so it was hard to understand why everyone wanted me to keep trying while saying that I wasn't improving. I fully admit that I wanted to stop taking my medications, but I had promised my mother that I wouldn't. My irrational idea of honor was the only thing that kept me medicated. Although I hated my medications, I do believe things would have become much worse had I not continued. To anyone reading this, I feel I must say that listening to my doctors saved my life.

On Valentine's Day that year I had no date and had cycled back into another depression. When I received a cute card from Nicoal, I wasn't even able to e-mail and thank her. Even though the card had not magically pulled me out of a depression, it did make me feel better. Over the next three months, I had a few weeks when I was somewhat normal. These times of normality had become more dreaded by my family than my swings, mostly because they had no way of knowing what might trigger a depressive or manic state. Looking back, I view living with me as like trying to run a sprint while holding nitroglycerine. My family never knew when I would explode.

When I received an e-mail from Nicoal telling me that she was flying back to Colorado to work during her summer vacation, I was eager to see her and was just beginning to enter my first and most mild stage of mania. I called her two days after she had returned, pleased to catch her on the phone.

"Hi, Nicoal, it's Kirk. I was wondering if you wanted to get together in the next few days." I didn't know why I felt nervous calling, but she sounded pleased to hear from me.

"I wish I could, but I have to work." I asked when she had time, and she responded with, "I'm really not sure." I was getting the idea that she wasn't interested, so I stopped calling.

Two weeks later, Nicoal called me. "You told me you would call me, but two weeks go by without a single call. What's going on?"

I was surprised to hear the anger in her voice as I had believed she was not interested in getting together. Knowing that Nicoal wasn't as experienced with dating as I, I just went with it. "I'm sorry. Honestly, you seemed really busy, and I didn't want to bother you."

"I've been working two jobs, but I was still looking forward to seeing you. I even have today off."

"Okay then. How does dinner sound?" I asked, deciding that if she wanted to see me and had the day off, I'd take the risk. "If you're free, I'll drive up. How about I pick you up at five?"

Nicoal paused, and heard surprise in her voice as she answered. "Okay. I'll see you then."

The moment I hung up the phone, I rushed to get ready and clean up. Leaving a note for my family since no one was home, I took my car keys and headed out.

When I picked up Nicoal, she was wearing a black dress decorated with a few sparkles. She was tan from her time in Florida attending college, but her black hair, gentle brown eyes, and dress matched well with her skin. Unlike last time, we were both aware that this was an official date, and for some reason things seemed harder than I remembered. After dinner, as we were walking back to the car, I was wondering if I had been wrong about the spark Nicoal and I had. When we reached the car and I opened the door for her, though, she embraced me with a long kiss. Suddenly the sparks were back, and the tension was gone. We both had been trying to force things when there was no need. This was the beginning of our real relationship.

As my mania continued to grow, Nicoal and I spent as much time as we could together. After only three weeks of dating, I knew I loved her. It wasn't the mania, although I believe I moved faster because of my mania. The love I felt was warm and different. When the summer came to a close, I was foolish enough to go to a jewelry store, bringing in my own design for an engagement ring. My family liked Nicoal, and everything seemed so easy, but I maxed out my credit card buying her a ring that I couldn't afford. Lost again in the present, I didn't wonder about Nicoal saying no to a marriage proposal. I just assumed she would say yes. Why wouldn't she? The fact she was only nineteen or that she was going back to Florida for school never even made me wonder.

When the summer was over, I approached her parents, asking for their blessings for me to propose. With Nicoal being so young, neither her mother nor father was entirely eager about the idea. Had they not given me their blessings, I would still have proposed to Nicoal. Luckily, after I answered some tough questions, they gave me their blessings. Bipolar destroyed my relationships and left my life in ruins on many occasions, and it was because of my mania that I asked a nineteen-year-old to marry me. With no degree or source of income, I was not thinking clearly. I was lost in the moment, unable to separate my present desires and emotions from reality and logic. My mania led to the single greatest risk I would ever take.

III.   CARING ENOUGH TO SEE THE TRUTH

When Nicoal left for Florida at the end of the summer, we decided that we would remain exclusive. I had tried a long-distance relationship before, but this time I thought it could work. There is a very good reason that many long-distance relationships don't work out, but in our case, it was probably the best possible situation for our relationship.

First of all, Nicoal never saw me struggle, so her idea of me and the reality of who I was were very different than the truth. It was not that I wanted to hide anything, but I still felt like I was fine and there was no need to scare Nicoal off with a story of me being bipolar. Second, I don't think she would ever have agreed to marry me had she seen how I really was. So in November 2002, despite my family's nervousness and Dr. Smith's strong objections, I proposed.

Although her parents had given me their blessings, they were worried about Nicoal making such a big decision at her age. Had they known that I was neither financially or mentally stable, they would never have let their daughter marry me, and I can't say that I would've blamed them. Luckily, however, things went smoothly, and Nicoal said yes.

The next time Nicoal was in town, her family wanted to celebrate our engagement. Nicoal and I drove together, meeting her family in Estes Park. Had I been able to sense my moods, I wouldn't have put myself in such a situation, for my mania was getting stronger. Not only was I snappy, aggressive, and out of sorts during the drive but I wasn't in the mood to socialize with Nicoal's family. I liked them, but I was craving excitement and a club, not a small mountain town.

As we were eating at the Stanley Hotel, Nicoal's mother noticed my hands shaking and kept asking if I was feeling well. The hand tremors that were caused by my medications had grown worse, but I simply lied and said I must have had too much caffeine. Neither one of her parents seemed to buy my excuse, but they let it go. After lunch, Nicoal's mom wanted to go shopping. Although I was beginning to feel anxious and a bit delusional, I couldn't say no.

When we arrived at the first store, I realized that I had forgotten my sunglasses at the hotel. They were expensive, so I was extremely angry with myself. Picking up that I was upset, Nicoal calmly walked over to me and touched my shoulder. "What is wrong, sweetie?"

"I left my glasses at the hotel," I said with disgust and anger. In my mind, I didn't want to have to go back and look, figuring I wouldn't find them.

"Why don't we just go back and get them?" Nicoal's suggestion was simple and logical, and it would've been easy, but I had slipped beyond seeing reason at that point.

"Someone probably already stole them," I said, my voice rising with anger as my mind took a small problem and blew it out of proportion. "I can't believe that I would forget them. Son of a …" As I was shouting, making a scene, Nicoal quickly pulled me out of the store and away from her parents who hadn't noticed my outburst.

Gently holding my hand and guiding me out to the street so we could talk, Nicoal spoke quietly. "You don't need to yell."

Pulling my hand away from hers, I knew I didn't need to yell, but I wanted to. "I can't believe you are giving me a hard time. I loved those glasses."

"So let's go get them."

"I can't believe we have to drive back! Damn it!" My anger and frustration made perfect sense to me, but to Nicoal, my reaction seemed more than odd as she looked at me with an odd expression.

"Are you feeling okay? Did my family upset you or something?" Nicoal was trying to understand why I was growing so angry, but there was no way she could. No sane individual could fathom the swirling thoughts in my head, nor understand why such a small thing could cause so much rage.

"I'm feeling fine. Just back off, okay!" My words were harsh and loud enough to make the other tourists nearby look over with the same curiosity that makes people slow down to see the scene of an accident. I hadn't noticed, but while I continued to curse in anger and walk down the street, Nicoal had run back inside the store to tell her parents we'd be right back. When she caught up to me, I wasn't myself. Although that day and what happened is one of my worst memories, it is also the point in time when I can clearly see my life's path change. Sometimes it takes losing or nearly losing something amazing to see the truth.

As we walked toward my parents' car, Nicoal was trying to calm me down, her voice soft as she spoke. "Kirk, I can just go get them if you don't want to go back. Do you want me to drive?"

Pulling the keys to my dad's Passat from my pocket and handing them to Nicoal, I spoke harshly to her. "I don't feel like driving. If you want to go back so badly, you drive." Nicoal did not deserve to be talked to the way I was speaking, nor did any person.

As we walked across a small bridge that spanned over a mountain river, Nicoal kept pressing me because she was worried. "You're not acting like you're okay. Just tell me. Did I upset you? You're so angry."

I snapped, my voice booming into the mountain air as Nicoal's gentle question sparked a huge argument. I had lost all control, and we shouted back and forth. During our fight, a tall man interrupted us, his deep voice sounding as he addressed me. "What is your problem?"

My rage quickly changed its focus as I turned, facing the tall man in his thirties. Although he was concerned about Nicoal, he had no idea what he was stepping into. "I'm trying to have a conversation with my fiancée, if you don't mind."

"I do mind, and how dare ..." the man was unable to finish as I reached out, grabbing him by his jacket and slamming him against the side of the bridge. I was lost to reality, unable to see the fear in his eyes as I held him over a long drop into the rushing river below.

"Stay the hell out of my way and business." I wasn't sure if I was shouting or growling, but I wanted to toss the man over the bridge—and might have had Nicoal not raised her voice.

"Let him go, Kirk," Nicoal said, her voice somehow cutting through my rage long enough for the man to slip out of my grasp before darting away.

As I continued to hold the bridge's metal railing with a tight grip, my anger roaring through me, Nicoal called my mother from her cell phone. She was worried about her parents seeing me in my current state and thought my mother might know how to calm me down. "Okay, I'll be careful," I heard her say before hanging up the phone.

"What did she tell you?"

Nicoal didn't answer as she as she hung up the phone, walking quickly to my side and saying, "Let's get to the car, now."

There was no doubt that I loved Nicoal, but when I met her eyes, there was a brief moment of clarity where I saw the horror she felt, making me wonder if she could ever see me the way I wanted her to again. My brief moment of clarity vanished as we moved quickly to the car, Nicoal's expression worried as tears streamed down her face.

Reaching the car without the keys, I felt an uncontrollable need to flee. Not because I was worried about someone calling the police, but because I wanted to run from what I had glimpsed in Nicoal's eyes. Seeing my reflection in the window of the passenger side of the car was too much for me to take, so I lashed out, hitting the window, luckily not hard enough to break it or my hand.

"Why don't we go for a short drive?" Nicoal said as she unlocked the doors.

I didn't realize it at the time, but Nicoal was trying to get me out of the area, especially as police sirens echoed through the small mountain town's sky. My actions had horrified not just Nicoal but everyone who had been watching. "I think we should go get your glasses," Nicoal said, a bit of panic in her voice.

If it had been any other person, I wouldn't have listened, but for some reason I opened the door and sat down—though not without slamming the door as hard as I could. The impact of the door shook the car and startled Nicoal. I continued to lash out, reaching up and pulling down on the handle above the passenger-side window until it snapped with a loud pop. Nicoal made a small squeaking sound as her shock was too great to hold in.

"Well, are we going or not?" I shouted, unable to see that I had hurt Nicoal in a way I might not be able to repair. For a brief moment, I actually wondered whether there truly was something wrong with me. It was the first time I had thought such a thing during a manic peak.

As Nicoal drove out of the parking lot, carefully avoiding the bridge where I had physically assaulted a total stranger, she sobbed. I clenched my fists as hard as I could. Unable to control the rage and frustration that were consuming my thoughts, I watched helplessly as the tears rolled down Nicoal's face. Suddenly, a single thought penetrated my fog of rage: *I'm going to lose her.* The brief moment of clarity was quickly torn away by my mania and rage.

That single moment of clarity, knowing I could lose Nicoal, is what propelled me to research bipolar and forever change my life. Love led me to the happiness and hope I now enjoy, and love is one of the many reasons I am now writing this memoir.

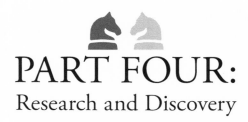

PART FOUR:
Research and Discovery

:: When Madness Helps ::

I.   TAKING ADVANTAGE OF MY MANIA

When I lost control in Estes Park, spewing hate-filled rhetoric and obscenities at the world, myself, and the woman I wanted to marry, it wasn't the first time my mania had overtaken my ability to think logically. Had Nicoal not been there to stop me, I have no doubt I would've thrown the tall stranger off the bridge.

It is horrifying to think of all the people I hurt, the damage I caused to property, or the beatings I took that I most surely deserved. Somehow, through some strange luck, I had always managed to avoid being arrested. There is little doubt that when my mania took over, there were many times when I should've been. When I was at my peak, lashing out, the fact that I believed I was acting out of self-preservation did not excuse my actions. In every outburst, I was always trapped in the present, my actions guided by my mania and the false realities it created.

What still startles me about Estes is that unlike during most of my manic outbursts, where I was unaware of and uncaring about my actions, seeing the pain I had caused in Nicoal's gentle eyes sent a ripple through my reality. Although it only lasted for a brief moment, it allowed me, for the first time in my life, to see beyond the thick veil of denial that kept me from seeing the truth. For a split second I had known that something was wrong. Although that day remains one of my worst memories, it is also the day that changed my life in ways that I am finally able to describe.

No longer shielded by the denial that had kept me from committing to my therapy or even believing that something might be wrong with me, I realized that I had no choice but to change. The problem, however, was that my bipolar was still in total control. Coming to terms with my mental illness did not change the fact that there was no cure or that the massive amount of medication I was taking still couldn't calm the ferocity of my swings.

At first I had believed that knowing the truth might have offered me a chance to take control, but the fact that I didn't want to be depressed or manic did not enhance my ability to overcome whatever current episode I was entrenched in. Feeling powerless without the ability to control myself, I hated the world more than ever.

No one who suffers from bipolar wants to feel the dark and ominous depression that makes life feel heavy, tireless, and meaningless, nor does anyone enjoy the anxiousness, paranoia, or delusions that accompany a manic episode. I was no different. Even after I knew that something was wrong, I had no ability to take control of my own mind or moods, making me feel powerless and trapped.

Although I hadn't been officially diagnosed until I was in college, it was becoming clear to me and my family that bipolar had long ago made me a passenger in my own life, not a pilot. Feeling like I was watching my life pass by, instead of feeling or living it, grew harder to take. I couldn't live as I was, and although I was delusional at the time, I was determined to find a way to calm my wild mind.

That night after we returned to Nicoal's house, Nicoal kept her distance from me. I could hear her parents asking if everything was all right as I hid in the spare bedroom, still angry as my mind raced. I wasn't about to go downstairs and eat with Nicoal's parents and sister as I couldn't shake the rage that controlled me. When Nicoal came up, I was already in bed, and she smiled at me gently. "Are you feeling better?"

"I'm fine," I responded—a response that Nicoal always hated.

"Okay," she said, not wanting to push me to talk about what had happened that day. Although she didn't talk, I could tell she was worried. She had watched me nearly kill another human being for no reason other than he came between us. Today, I know the only reason she didn't run was because of her own past and the horrors she had seen. "Good night," she added, kissing me on the cheek before crawling into bed next to me, wrapping her arms around me. I wanted to reach out and hold Nicoal, but I remained still and cold, staring up at the ceiling fan that spun slowly above the guest room's bed.

Nicoal eventually fell asleep while I, on the other hand, spent the night trying to slow down my racing mind. For a long while I thought about telling Nicoal that I was bipolar, but I was afraid of losing her. I also knew that her parents wouldn't hear of their daughter marrying someone with bipolar. Although I did not think they would judge me, I was well aware of how protective they were of their daughter. It didn't take me long to decide that I wouldn't tell Nicoal. I would get better first and then tell her. I can see now how selfish I was being, but in my defense, at that time, I was still manic and was unable to see how my actions could affect others.

As I felt my rage turning to energy that I needed and wanted to burn off, I looked down, seeing Nicoal's arms around me. For a very brief moment, I felt at peace. Nicoal was heading back to Florida in the morning, and although I was sad to see her go, I knew what I needed to do.

The morning came quickly, Nicoal waking up to find me dressed and ready to take her to the airport. As if sleep had made my actions sink into Nicoal's mind, she looked at me cautiously, unsure how I would be feeling. Had she been as mentally strong as she is now, I have no doubt she would've left me long before we exchanged vows. In a crazy way, we were both mentally hindered, giving us a chance to grow and heal together.

Kissing at the security gate and saying good-bye, I asked her to call when she arrived safely. With that, we parted, a new doubt cast upon our relationship. As I walked out of the airport and into the parking garage, I kept thinking about the first time I had met Dr. Smith. He had said that there was no cure to bipolar and warned me that I might not ever be able to lead a normal life. Opening the door to the car, I whispered under my breath, "He's wrong."

Since I had yet to reach the peak of my mania, I drove home, ready to prove the world wrong. I was finally willing to admit that something was wrong with my mind, but I wasn't ready to admit that I could do nothing about it.

Arriving at my house, I walked in with a mission. My mother, pacing in front of the door, was worried after receiving the previous day's phone call from Nicoal. My little explosion in Estes had worried everyone, but my mom could tell I was on the move and simply let me head down to my room.

For the next week, I slept a few hours here and there, but when awake I was lost in research. The more I read about bipolar, the more the veil of denial faded away. As Dr. Smith had said, I had a textbook case of bipolar I. Misguided by an elevated sense of my own abilities, I feel quite comfortable calling myself a mad scientist during my research. One thing bothered me as I researched. Every single blog, medical journal, book, or memoir said that the key to treating bipolar was staying on medication and that most of the extreme cases studied were never able to function, regardless of their medication. As with other extreme cases, my medications weren't curing my ills or making my swings better. I have no idea how badly off I would've been without them, but I wanted more than the life I was currently living: I wanted a cure.

After I spent a week researching every medication and treatment for bipolar disorder, my mania began to peak, and my ability to research or focus vanished. I was a bit delusional when I shut off my computer, swearing that everyone was wrong. There had to be a cure, and I was determined to find it. Moreover, I believed I could actually do it. I didn't know that I would eventually stumble onto something that would forever change my life.

Unable to concentrate, I stood up and looked around my room, which was littered with large stacks of printed articles, medical studies, and journals that I had highlighted and studied in a desperate attempt to find answers or holes that would lead me to an answer. While in my beginning two stages of mania, I became obsessed as my understanding of bipolar, the brain, and medications deepened. The only problem was that everything I found pointed to the same answer: there was no cure.

Eventually, I had to research beyond the narrow scope of bipolar, still convinced that someone had missed something. Only a delusional fool would've thought he could cure something that wasn't curable. The irony is that without mania to drive my research, I would not be the man I am today.

Although it took me several years, I finally found a different approach to looking at bipolar and its method of treatment. I never quit taking my medication, but I did begin experimenting on myself as only a madman would. There are reasons for the ethical and scientific guidelines that direct how medical studies and tests are performed, but I was not a doctor, and I was hardly sane. Living in the present, desperate to find a cure while feeling indestructible, I took chances that nearly killed me.

Somehow, through a mixture of research, luck, and a willingness to risk life and limb on a scientifically based hunch, I discovered a new method of treating my bipolar. My discovery not only led to my complete recovery, which has left me free of bipolar for over five years, but also proves that there is always hope.

I must say again that although I was foolish enough to experiment on myself, I do not condone such actions. Anyone suffering from bipolar should listen to and work with a medical professional. Whoever reads this must understand that changing medications or experimenting nearly killed me and did cause lasting damage that I will have to deal with for the remainder of my life.

II.   FAILING HEALTH AND THE CONTINUED SEARCH FOR ANSWERS

During my research it became very clear that I did, in fact, have an extreme case of bipolar. It was a strange experience to feel as if I was perfectly normal and yet know, deep down, that something was terribly wrong. Researching bipolar and all its medications and treatments helped by making my mental disorder less personal and more scientific, but understanding and accepting my condition didn't make the disorder better. The more I read, the more committed I became to my medications and even my therapy. I had not yet discovered anything, so I was trying my best to stick with my current medications, seeking therapy, and even trying group support.

Wanting to improve and actually getting better were two very different things. The harder I tried to calm myself and recognize my moods, the more I felt like no amount of effort would ever lead to control or normality. This became increasingly infuriating. No matter how hard I tried, the swings still came, my manic days filled with research and their peaks ending with drug use and a crash into depression.

My bipolar was continuing to control my life, and when my mania wasn't sharpening my mind and speeding the world and reality around me, I felt sluggish, dim, and stupid. The side effects of my daily medications continued to get worse, and countless times I would walk upstairs only to wonder why I had come upstairs in the first place. My balance and vision were also affected, and I began to trip and walk into walls occasionally. I even fell down the stairs once, crashing through the drywall and cracking two wooden studs with my weight and momentum. However, what concerned my family more than the side effects was that my physical health was also beginning to deteriorate. I kept researching when I could, refusing to believe that my fate was not my own.

After moving down from the mountains to Denver, I had found a great doctor whom I trusted completely. When Dr. Smith wasn't monitoring my blood levels, Dr. Simon took care of me. Dr. Simon was one of the smartest doctors I had ever worked with and was utterly devoted to his work. I was lucky to have him, and, more importantly, I felt like I could confide in him. When my stomach problems, which I had struggled with my entire life, became bad enough that the first thing I looked for when walking into a building was a bathroom, my mother made an appointment for me to see Dr. Simon. It had been quite some time since I had seen a doctor for any reason other than bipolar.

After we walked into his small waiting room, my mother motioned for me to take a seat as she signed me in. I plopped down in the corner, trying to keep as much distance from everyone as I could. Everyone's voices seemed loud, and I ached all over. I had recently crashed from a manic peak and wanted nothing more than to be home, escaping the world around me with the aid of sleep.

"Kirk Miller," called a kind nurse named Suzie. Suzie saw me and opened the door to the hallway filled with examination rooms. "You're at the end, Kirk," Suzie said gently. Quickly seeing that I was not feeling well, she was about to come and help me to my feet when I felt my mother help lift me, guiding me past Suzie. My stomach was aching again and hurt enough that moving was hard.

Suzie followed us to the last exam room, closing the door behind us as my mother helped me sit down on the exam table covered with a light pink fabric and paper that crackled when I sat down. Seeing that I didn't feel well enough to stand back up for her to check my height and weight, Suzie pulled out her pen and began asking her normal questions. "Are you at the same weight?" When I nodded, she continued. "What medications are you taking?"

It is hard to look at the past, knowing that I wasn't even aware of how much of each medication I was taking. I was also oblivious to the dosage. Had I been living on my own like most men at the age of twenty-four, I'm not sure I would've been able to keep track of my medications.

Seeing that I had no idea, my mother answered for me. "He's taking the same dosage of lithium, clonazepam, Lamictal, and Synthroid as on our last visit."

"What about any other medications?"

"Dr. Smith took him off the antipsychotic since it didn't seem to be helping, but other than that, nothing has changed."

After taking my temperature and blood pressure, Suzie returned to her clipboard, asking, "So why are we seeing you today?"

"I'm having some stomach issues." Before Suzie could ask me what kind of issues, I followed up my statement with, "I'd prefer to talk about it with Dr. Simon." It wasn't that I was embarrassed, but I felt more comfortable talking about my bowel movements to a guy. It was bad enough that my family had noticed my problem.

"Okay then." Suzie nodded, opening the door and sliding my file into the wooden slot resting on the front of the door. "Dr. Simon will be with you in a jiffy."

Since Dr. Simon had delivered me and my sister and had known my mother for a long time, he had made room for us in his closed practice. I didn't go to him because we had history; I went to him, as did my family, because he was the best doctor we had ever dealt with.

An older man with gray hair, Dr. Simon was always dressed in a suit and red tie. The outfit was topped off by the expensive stethoscope that always hung around his neck. He had grown up in the days before people understood how dangerous smoking was, so his voice, although warm and gentle, had a bit of a rasp to it as he greeted my mother. "Hi, Jeanne," he said warmly before turning to face me. He took one look at me and stated, "You don't look so good."

Looking down at the chart, he quickly looked at all my numbers before asking, "So what's the problem with your stomach?"

"I'm going to the bathroom a lot."

"What do you mean by 'a lot'?" Dr. Simon asked. "A number or a guess would help me out."

Although I was trying to eat healthily, I was going to the bathroom at least ten times or more a day, so I told him, "Over ten times per day."

My mother interjected, "Every time we go somewhere, the first thing he looks for is a bathroom, and some days it is far more than ten times."

Dr. Simon just nodded. "Well, I'd say that's more trips than a young one like yourself should be making. Can you lie back?" I did as I was told as Dr. Simon came and pressed on my stomach, making small circles with his fingertips. As he was examining me, he turned to my mother and asked, "What have you tried?" Dr. Simon knew that my father was a pharmacist and was smart enough to assume that we had tried as much as we could before visiting him.

My mother listed off vitamins and probiotics and then a few medications that made Dr. Simon's smile begin to fade. Although he was an older man, his eyes were sharp, and you could almost see the man thinking as my mother added, "We've tried everything, but nothing seems to help."

Dr. Simon stopped pressing on my stomach and stepped back. "You can sit up," he said, waiting for me to do so before asking, "What do your stools look like?" Dr. Simon had a way of making even the most embarrassing questions seem harmless, so I answered.

"I usually have diarrhea." After I answered a few more questions, explaining the constant pain and urgency to go to the bathroom, Dr. Simon appeared to have made up his mind.

"I think it would be wise to schedule a colonoscopy, but in the meantime, I'm going to prescribe Prednisone." Seeing my mom's eyes widen at the mention of the drug, I was curious.

Although I didn't feel like a conversation, I did want to know. "And what is Prednisone?"

"It's a powerful steroid that is commonly used to treat inflammation. I'm only giving you a small dose for a few days, so keep a close eye on your improvement."

"Steroid?"

Dr. Simon smiled, knowing exactly what I was thinking. "Prednisone is a corticosteroid, not an anabolic steroid like you hear about in the media. I think you have irritable bowel syndrome, and although Prednisone isn't my first choice, it sounds like your dad has already tried all my preferred options. Your problem is severe enough that we'll give Prednisone a chance and see how you do. You only have enough for five days, so we'll reevaluate in a week." With that, Dr. Simon wrote me a prescription and said good-bye to my mother before he stepped out of the room, always the professional.

"And yet another pill." I had spoken quietly, but my mother caught my words. Concerned, she walked over and gave me a hug. Looking down at the prescription, I said exactly what I was thinking, "I'm tired of this, Mom."

"I know you are, sweetie. Let's go."

With that, we walked out of the exam room and drove back home. Stopping at the pharmacy nearest to our house, we sat and waited for the pharmacist to fill the Prednisone prescription. My gut and stomach were churning. The only way I could lessen my pain was to lean forward and clutch my stomach. My stomach ached badly enough that I was actually looking forward to taking the medication that Dr. Simon had prescribed. It was beyond my ability to feel optimistic as my life, and now my body, fell apart. Luckily, Nicoal and I were still together, our plans unchanged even after my manic episode.

When the pharmacist handed us the prescription, my mother opened the bag and the bottle before handing me a single pill. As Dr. Simon had instructed, I took the pill from my mother's hand and plopped it into my mouth. I had become so used to taking pills that I no longer needed water.

When I awoke the next morning, my stomach still ached, but it wasn't as bad as it usually was. My depression, however, had grown more severe and had done so more quickly than in the past. Although my stomach was feeling a bit better, my mind was a wreck. I wanted to stay in bed and sleep, but my thirst and need to relieve my bladder were enough to get me moving.

Rolling to my side and swinging my legs over the edge of the bed, I sat for a long moment, my head down and my hands pressed down against the side of the bed. Even as small slits of sun came in through my window, everything felt dark to me. The colors of the posters on my wall looked dim again, and I had no idea how I would face another day.

Sighing, I reached up to my eyes, rubbing them gently because they itched. The moment my hands touched my face, I paused. Something wasn't right. Gently running my fingers over my face, I could feel small bumps covering my skin. Wondering what was going on, I forced myself out of bed and walked into my bathroom. I should've felt a sense of panic, but the bleakness of my worldview overpowered my normal thought process.

When I flicked the bathroom lights on and looked into my mirror, my eyes widened. My entire body was covered with small bumps that looked like sunburn blisters. Reaching up with my right index finger, I touched one. The blister was so soft that it broke open, releasing a clear liquid. I remember shrugging my shoulders and deciding that I must have had some allergic reaction that sleep would cure.

As I turned away from the mirror, planning on returning to my bedroom, I saw my mother standing in the doorway holding a tray covered with breakfast foods. When she saw the blisters covering my body, her eyes widened, and she nearly dropped the tray she was holding.

Quickly setting down the food, my mother rushed to my side. "What happened?" she asked, her shock quieting her voice as it came out more like a whisper. Her whisper quickly changed as she turned away from me and shouted loudly enough that it made me cringe. "Jackson!"

I heard my dad's feet running down the stairs above me. It was Friday, and my dad had just happened to have the day off. "Mom, it's not a big deal. Just let me go back to bed." I tried to move past her, but she held her ground. I didn't have the energy to argue, so I backed up and leaned against the edge of my sink.

Rushing down the stairs so fast that he nearly tripped over the food on the stairs, my dad ran into the bathroom with wide eyes. My mom's shout had startled him, to say the least. "What's wrong?" Seeing that there was no major emergency, my father took a breath of relief as my mom pointed at my face. When it came to medical issues, my father never panicked. To me, my father had always seemed more like a doctor than a pharmacist, always knowing what illness we had before it was confirmed by a test or a doctor. I had always respected his medical opinions, so I just sighed and let him come close enough to take a look. "Looks like sunburn blisters," he mumbled to himself before stepping back and adding, "Are the blisters anywhere else?"

"I just woke up. How would I know?"

"Kirk Patrick," my mother said, using my middle name as she always did when she was upset with me, "Please don't talk to your father like that." The truth was that despite how much I respected and loved my father, I never spoke to him with respect. I was usually very short and impatient with him without any good reason.

"Fine," I retorted as I stripped off my shirt. "Are you both happy now?" When I saw my mother's face turn pale and my father's eyes shimmer with surprise, I looked down. The blisters not only were on my face but also ran down my arms, chest, back, stomach, and even legs.

"Dr. Simon is out of the office today, Jackson. What should we do?" my mother asked, panicked and on the verge of tears as she looked pleadingly to my father.

As always, my dad remained calm. "There is no reason to panic, although I'm not sure what the blisters are. We need to get to a dermatologist."

"Another freakin' doctor," I said, throwing up my hands. "Wouldn't it be easier if someone just shot me?"

I didn't realize at the time how dark my statement was, but apparently it was the final straw. Concern filled my father's eyes, and my mother rushed out of the bathroom, upset that I would say such a thing.

"You shouldn't talk like that," my father said quietly as he examined my blisters. "It upsets your mother, and, to be frank, I don't like it either." Before I could respond, he asked, "Did you eat anything different yesterday?"

"No, but I did start taking Prednisone."

"That's strange. If anything, I would expect that the Prednisone would have helped the blisters. I don't think it could cause this." Reaching up, he touched my face where I had popped one of the blisters. "Now that is odd."

When he pulled back his hand, he held his finger up to the light so that I could see. The liquid that had come out of my blister had dried, turning into what looked like an amber crystal. "Looks like dermatitis herpetiformis, but does it itch?"

"No," I responded, making my dad pause and reflect.

"It isn't related to the Lamictal, but I still don't like it."

Putting my shirt back on and feeling some of the blisters on my back break as the T-shirt slid across them, I might have found humor in how complex my body was if I weren't so despondent. I was already heading out of the bathroom and toward my bedroom when I felt my mother take hold of my wrist.

"What?" I asked, about to pull away when she answered.

"Get dressed. We have an appointment in thirty minutes."

I had not expected my mom to be able to get an appointment with a dermatologist, especially on the same day that she called, but when push came to shove there wasn't much my mom couldn't do. She rushed me out the door after giving me my daily handful of pills. We got into the car, and my mom took off, driving fast enough that our thirty-minute drive only took twenty.

Walking into the building, my mother pointed to the large waiting area and said, "You just go sit down and relax. I'll fill everything out."

Seeing a large fish tank in the center of the waiting room, I walked toward the tank and sat down. Watching the fish darting through the fake coral and plants in the tank, I sighed. I felt worthless. Unable to hold a job, terrifying my family and Nicoal with my swings, I just wasn't prepared for my body to begin failing.

A blanket of dark thoughts suddenly enveloped my mind. I hated feeling so vulnerable and pathetic. Just as I was about to close my eyes, a nurse called my name. I would learn years later that the only reason they had agreed to see me was because my mother had caused a stir. There is no force as strong as a protective and loving mother. That I now take as simple fact.

After a nurse showed me to a large and high-tech exam room with bright paintings and light that hurt my eyes, she quickly took down my medical history before pressing a small red button on the wall and saying, "Dr. Wright will be with you in a moment."

"Dr. Simon told me that Dr. Wright was the best dermatologist he knew," my mother said in an attempt to lighten my mood, adding, "I'm sure it's nothing."

Dr. Wright walked in a few moments later. At first he seemed a bit annoyed as we had forced our way into an appointment, but his annoyance quickly changed to curiosity when he saw my face and neck. Dr. Wright was a tall man in a neatly pressed lab coat that matched the white hair lining the sides of his bald head. His thick, square glasses made his eyes look comically large, but he was all about business. Without a word, he sat down on his stool, rolling toward me as he touched and examined my blisters with gloved hands. Rolling back and pressing the intercom button, Dr. Wright spoke in a sharp and commanding voice. "I need surgical equipment for a biopsy in exam room six."

I knew what a biopsy was, so I took off my shirt so he could choose a less obvious place to take a small skin sample. As a nurse came into the room with a tray of surgical tools, I had to ask. "What do you think it is?"

Dr. Wright shook his head. "It looks much like dermatitis herpetiformis, which is very treatable, but this is all over your body, which is strange. That's why I'm going to take two biopsies, one to send to a university and one for our lab. If this is how your skin reacted after taking Prednisone, than I'd like to make sure we know what is going on so that we treat it properly."

It was a good answer, and I didn't have the energy to argue, so I took off my shirt and lay back on the table. Dr. Wright took two biopsies from the center of my chest while setting up an appointment for the following week. After he stitched up one of the larger cuts and left the room, I put my shirt on and sighed. "Can we go home?" I asked.

I don't know how I must have sounded, but my mother's entire face fell. "Of course, sweetie."

One week later, I was back in the same examination room, totally unaware of the bad news I was about to receive.

Most of my blisters had faded away, but many still remained. Since my depression had moved into its second stage, I was having extremely dark thoughts. Not feeling like I could go out in public due to my blisters only made me hate everything with a higher intensity. It took both my sister and mother to get me out of bed, dressed, and into the car so that I could make my appointment with Dr. Wright.

Once at the doctor's office, my sister came to the passenger side door, opening it and reaching out to take hold of my hand. "Kirken," she said, using the name my family often called me by, "let's get you into that office so you can enjoy the rest of the day." As always, my sister was trying her hardest to smile and help keep my mother from breaking down into tears.

When my sister got me out of the car, I held on to her tiny frame, feeling weak and tired as we walked into the doctor's office and eventually the exam room. I was still taking the Prednisone along with all my other medications, as Dr. Wright, Dr. Simon, and my father all figured it would help, but I was getting only minute relief from my stomach problems, and now my skin had caused a new problem. As I sat in the exam room, I truly believed that my family would be better off without me. Such suicidal thoughts had become common over the last few days and not knowing what was wrong with my skin had only made me feel that much more useless. Luckily, although I had every intention to end my own life, by the time I wanted to, I was too depressed and tired to act. Had I been just a bit happier or energized, or even on an antidepressant, I know I would have taken my life.

My sister sat next to me on the exam table, patting my back as we waited to hear what the results of my tests were. When the door opened, Dr. Wright entered the room in the same way as before, but this time he took the time to introduce himself to us all before examining my blisters once more. "The tests came back, and you have what is referred to as Linear IGA dermatosis. It is an incredibly rare autoimmune disease that causes blistering just beneath the skin. Had we not sent it to the university, I doubt we would have figured it out so quickly."

I had been researching enough medical journals and studies that I knew exactly what an autoimmune disease was. To say that it was bad news was an understatement. Not only was my mind a disaster but my own immune system was attacking itself. "So what's the treatment?" my sister asked. I already figured I'd need more pills, and I wasn't wrong.

"Well." Dr. Wright paused and took a deep breath before continuing. "Usually, we would give a corticosteroid to control your current outburst, but it isn't a good long-term treatment, and you're already taking Prednisone, which should have suppressed your blisters in the first place. The long-term solution that I would suggest is taking a drug called Dapsone."

Dr. Wright explained that I would need to have regular blood tests so that they could make sure the Dapsone wasn't causing major damage, especially with my combination of other drugs. Had I been able, I would've laughed at the idea of being on another medication that had the potential to kill me. The appointment flew by, and before I knew it I was back home and my mother had added yet another drug to my long list of medications.

Luckily, after taking the Dapsone my blisters cleared right up. Although I would always have Linear IGA and the autoimmune issue, at least my body wasn't covered with blisters as well. I would be on Dapsone for the rest of my life, however. When Dr. Simon heard about what had happened with the Prednisone, he was as stumped as Dr. Wright had been. He was not happy about pulling me off the Prednisone, which had finally begun to help my stomach, but he had not liked the reaction it had caused.

As usual, one problem seemed to lead to another, continuing to pile up and adding to my feeling that my family would be better off without me.

Two weeks later, even though my stomach pains returned, I was finally climbing out of my depression. After taking a long shower, shaving, and eating a small breakfast, I was in the mood to continue with my research. When I walked upstairs and into the kitchen to take my pills, I wasn't sure why my sister and mother seemed on edge. Of course, I didn't know that whenever I cleaned myself up, my mother and sister knew that the worst of my downs were gone and wondered when my mania would overtake me and if I would simply vanish one day. Their fears were very justified.

Taking my pills, I left the kitchen and headed down to my room with a bottle of water, ready to spend the day researching. I cleared my desk of all the medical journals and articles that I had read and marked, sat down in my comfortable chair, and turned to my computer. The moment I sat down, my stomach tightened up, and I bent over to lessen the pain. Although I could handle the pain, it was a bit harder because the Prednisone had given me a short taste of what it was like to live without the debilitating pain. In some ways, it would've been easier if I hadn't ever felt relief.

Frustrated at my options, I was convinced that there had to be something else that would act similarly to Prednisone. I was in enough pain that I set aside my research on bipolar and started looking into something that might help my IBS.

After a few days of researching for something that wasn't a corticosteroid but still had the anti-inflammatory benefits, I found an interesting study comparing the ability of cortisone and something called nandrolone decanoate. Research had analyzed and compared the two drugs, evaluating which was more beneficial in controlling inflammation and healing torn muscles in three groups of rats. Although the nandrolone decanoate was not as effective as the cortisone when it came to reducing inflammation, the drug still give far better results than the control group. Also, the rats that were given nandrolone decanoate had surpassed the control and cortisone groups in overall health by such a wide margin that I was stunned and fascinated.

Hence, I began my research into nandrolone decanoate. When I began my side research, I had no idea that nandrolone was an anabolic steroid or that its use was illegal without a written prescription. After a day of reading, I was amazed that the drug wasn't used more often. Not only did it have some anti-inflammatory benefits but it had also been shown to be incredibly helpful with many major diseases and injuries. Due to the stigma surrounding anabolic steroids, however, it was never talked about, and I knew no doctor would prescribe it for irritable bowel syndrome.

Had I been a sane individual and traditionally trained in medicine I would have discounted the use of nandrolone decanoate due to its legality. It did have side effects, but they were seen mostly on women and men taking higher-than-therapeutic doses. I wasn't sane and was certainly not shy about risks. After a bit more research, I decided I was going to take control of my own body. To say the least, this was my mania speaking, and was a terrible idea, but I didn't live in everyone else's world. I lived in my own, making my own rules, and breaking them was easy.

Over the next few months, I learned more about the compound nandrolone decanoate. Multiple studies from prestigious universities had used the drug to help patients with everything from AIDS to arthritis and lupus. As my mania kicked up, I acted, unaware that my life would forever be changed.

III.   DIVING HEADFIRST INTO SELF-EXPERIMENTATION

The more I researched all the medical uses for anabolic steroids, the more I was astounded that the use of such drugs was looked down upon by almost all medical professionals. I was aware that some individuals interested in increasing their athletic performance would abuse such drugs, but I couldn't fathom why the drugs themselves were not being applied more often in normal medical situations. Needless to say, it became all too clear that there wasn't a doctor on the planet who would write me a prescription for such a drug. As I continued to suffer from the pain my IBS caused, I did what I had always done when I wanted something but couldn't have it. I went around the law to procure what I desired.

Since I had more than enough connections in the illicit drug market, I made some calls and set up a meeting. The main problem with getting hold of nandrolone decanoate was that it was commonly counterfeited. Although none of my sources for drugs dealt anything like anabolic steroids, eventually I landed a solid connection.

After sending several coded messages by e-mail, I was given explicit instructions about where and how to send an amount of cash. A normal individual would've thought twice about sending cash in the mail, but I had been told that my source was well-known in steroid and athletic circles. By his standards, my order was small, but because he knew a mutual friend he decided to work with me.

I followed my source's instructions, and a package showed up at my house two weeks later. Thinking back, I can't believe I wasn't worried about someone finding my incoming package and opening it. Although my mother didn't usually open my mail, she did, on occasion, open something up by mistake. I did not want to explain what I had ordered, especially to my dad, who knew as well as I that even possessing anabolic steroids without a prescription was grounds for swift and severe punishment. Unable to see beyond my current need and the present, I never even thought about the ramifications of getting caught.

Home alone when the package was dropped off, I was excited to see what I had paid a few hundred dollars for. I carefully picked up the package, walked into my basement bathroom, shut the door behind me, and opened the package.

Inside, I counted twenty small boxes containing two-milliliter vials of nandrolone decanoate. The boxes were taped and packaged to avoid any damage during their shipment. Taking them out and setting them down, I returned to the box and retrieved the remainder of my order. Since I had been manic at the time I had placed my order, I had also ordered twenty glass ampoules of testosterone enanathate, which looked like light yellow baby oil. Lastly, I retrieved the twenty syringes I had ordered along with the medications. I knew where and how to inject the nandrolone decanoate, but I had expected small needles like the ones I had used before for drugs. These needles, however, were over an inch long, which should've made me nervous. Not even considering I could be making a mistake, I loaded a syringe, cleaned an area of my skin, and poked the long needle through my skin into the muscle. The fact that I never hesitated speaks to my desperation as well as my mental state. No normal person would be foolish enough to inject themselves without even a slight hint of fear. To me, it was time to take action and fix my body. I was tired of the doctors trying, and, being in my second stage of mania, I was foolish enough to think I knew better.

After removing the needle, I sat down and stared at the illegal drugs with a thin and dangerous smile across my lips. I had researched the proper dosages as well as how to properly administer the injectable esters, but that didn't change the fact that I was playing on a hunch, hoping the anabolic steroids would help my IBS as the Prednisone had.

With no way of knowing and no instant feeling from the injection, I shrugged and cleaned the droplet of blood from the injection site. Only looking back do I see the risks I was taking. Not only did I have enough of the substance to be held as a distributer but I also didn't even know if the stuff was real. Looking at the empty vial, I knew I had done my research. After taking the plunge, I knew it was now simply a waiting game.

Three days later, my stomach had not improved and my mania was growing in intensity. I had researched how anabolic steroids could affect bipolar, and every doctor and expert warned against using steroids; however, this wasn't about my bipolar. I couldn't research for something to help my bipolar when I was hunched over in pain all the time from my IBS.

I had carefully hidden all my drugs and syringes so that no one would discover them, but I was growing impatient. I was supposed to be feeling better, but I wasn't. The studies I had carefully read and researched had shown nandrolone decanoate to work as an anti-inflammatory while strengthening the bones and immune system, and so I wasn't pleased that I wasn't feeling better.

Angry that I wasn't better and not thinking straight due to my mania, I made a common mistake, thinking that if one vial didn't work, perhaps two or three would. That day I did three more injections, making my weekly dose of nandrolone more than four times the medical dose for males. I knew that it took time for the anabolic steroids to enter and affect my system, yet still I took the risk. Logic and knowledge could not compete with the power of my mania.

As the next few days went on, my skin blistered violently, and I had to double my dose of Dapsone to keep the blisters under control. I was supposed to do one injection a week, and it had already been five days, making me wonder if I should inject more. I had spent some time at the gym and hadn't noticed a difference in strength either, making me wonder if my contact had ripped me off.

When I awoke to the sound of my alarm the next day, I started to reach toward my eyes but stopped, realizing that my stomach, which was usually aching and churning after a night's sleep, was calm and painless. Laughing out loud, I lay in bed and ran my hands over my stomach before hitting the bed with both hands in celebration. Although I needed to release my bladder, I felt no pain and no urgency to go to the bathroom for the first time in months. Also, the extra dose of Dapsone must have helped, because my skin was clear of all blisters.

Still wondering if my contact had sent me the real steroid, I gave it a few days, each day my stomach feeling better and my skin clear. I was ready to get back to my bipolar research, not realizing what I had just accomplished.

That day, I decided I'd give my stomach a test, eating some fried food and candy that usually made my stomach worse. "Kirk," my mother said, seeing what I was about to eat. "You shouldn't eat that or it will upset your stomach."

"Not today," I said with a grin that made my mother's face fill with concern.

Not knowing what to expect, my mother simply touched my shoulder and added, "Just go slow, okay?"

I nodded, wanting to see if this was just a fluke or if I had been right. I had already decided that if the medication worked, I would be ordering more. Besides ordering more, I also knew that I wasn't going to start with two hundred milligrams. If the dose I was taking worked, I wasn't about to change it. Not only was I foolish but anyone who had studied androgenic anabolic steroids would have told me that I was taking far more than was medically necessary. Although the anabolic steroids weren't as expensive as the recreational drugs, they weren't cheap either. Had I been aware of myself, my mania, or my actions, I might have thought twice about trying a lower dose, if for no other reason than cost. At my current dose, I would be out of the nandrolone in four weeks. Luckily, now that my stomach was feeling better, I was able to take a few odd jobs when I needed cash. When my stomach stayed steady and calm even with all the food I had thrown at it, I began to widen my research to both bipolar and anabolic steroids.

For two weeks, my mania stayed steady, allowing me to gather a massive amount of information about anabolic steroids and bipolar. Most individuals who used the drugs recreationally would do what they called a "cycle," staying on the steroids for a certain amount of time before giving their body a rest. Anabolic steroids did have side effects, which I began to look into more deeply, not because I was worried but because of how many men and women reported having symptoms much like bipolar when coming on and off their cycles.

As I began to gain size and strength while weight training, my body weight also began to increase at a more dramatic rate than normal. No one in my family would have considered that I was taking anabolic steroids, so they just thought I was working out more consistently. Although my body was improving, my bipolar was still present. I continued to have swings of both depression and mania, yet I was feeling just a slight bit more stable. It certainly wasn't an amazing difference, but something had changed.

After six months of taking the anabolic steroids, I could sometimes see my moods, only now it wasn't just for a brief moment. My family had noticed that my swings were happening less often, and I had decided to try and start teaching the violin instead of just playing at events. I only had two students at the time, but I was able to handle them. Although I was still having swings, I began to realize that something positive was happening. I had been taking my bipolar drugs for over five years, but they had never made me as stable as I currently was. Therefore, I began to wonder if, against all odds and medical science, the anabolic steroids were helping me. I never told anyone what I was taking, but it was only a matter of time before I would have to tell Dr. Simon.

Nicoal finished her associate's degree and moved to Colorado to finish her business degree. Luckily, at the beginning of our real relationship, I tended to be more manic than depressed, but eventually I had no choice but to tell her that I had bipolar before getting married. I had been fearing the conversation, but when I told her, she simply shook her head and said something I will never forget: "No, you don't."

It was proof that love truly was blind. I was not easy to handle, and most women would not be strong enough to handle me when I couldn't handle myself.

The longer we lived together in my parents' basement, the more wild and explosive my actions became, making the truth apparent to her. When she confronted me about it, I swore to her that I was getting better. When I told her that, I realized that I had been completely truthful: I was getting better, even if at a slow pace.

I had gained around twenty-five pounds since I began injecting myself with anabolic steroids, not all of it muscle as the media would have people believe. I'm not saying that the anabolic steroids didn't help me gain muscle, but I wasn't working out consistently enough to utilize the large doses I was taking. However, because the steroids had calmed my IBS, for the first time in my life I found it easy to gain weight. I never thought that my large physique would raise some red flags when it was time for my annual physical.

My mother had scheduled an appointment with Dr. Simon for a time when she could go, as I still wasn't at the point where I could really take care of myself. Unlike during our usual visits to the doctor, I was in a good mood that day, joking with my mom as we drove down to Dr. Simon's office. I was doing better, and the entire family felt calmer.

There had been some setbacks; my last manic peak ended with me smashing every piece of scrap wood we had in our garage. Luckily, only my father had been home. More interesting, though, was that he had watched me the entire time, telling me that he thought I was getting better. He had noticed that I was selecting what I was hitting, as if deep down I was thinking of the value of what I was destroying. Although I dislike the memory, it is the first time that there was a visible change in my peaks. I didn't crash into a depression, so, overall, it was a huge difference.

When we walked into Dr. Simon's waiting room, my mother signed me in as I sat down, flipping through a magazine without really paying attention. Although I still had swings, everyone felt like I was far better than ever before. I waved my mother over and gestured to the seat next to mine. "Mom, you should read this article." I had no idea that even the way I was treating my mother was different. She cautiously walked over and sat next to me.

After about twenty minutes, Suzie called my name. I expected her to lead me to the same exam room we always had, but she stopped me and pointed to the scale, saying, "You've certainly bulked up since I last saw you."

"Lots of protein and working out," I said while stepping up on the scale. Since I didn't always have to go to the bathroom, I had been able to keep some weight on, and my strength had certainly improved.

Suzie had to adjust the scale, her face a bit surprised when the scale came to a balance. "So how much have I gained?" I asked after the scale came to a balance.

"Thirty-six pounds," Suzie said, her voice mixed with worry and surprise. "That's quite a bit of weight to pack on in eight months."

My mother smiled and said, "He's been at the gym more consistently, and his IBS is gone." She was obviously pleased that I was staying more stable, yet she had no idea that I was taking anything other than my bipolar medications, nor did anyone else.

Suzie led us to the last room, checking my temperature and asking her standard questions as she took my blood pressure. "Your blood pressure is high, but everything else seems fine. Dr. Simon will be with you in a moment."

Dr. Simon entered the room, wearing a sleek blue blazer and skinny red tie, and gave my mother a quick hug before turning toward me. When he saw me, his eyes sharpened, and he looked down at the chart. "So, how has your IBS been?"

"I've been doing really well," I responded, not sure how to explain that I had gone from having chronic pain and constant diarrhea to having a regular schedule. "No complaints here."

Dr. Simon looked at my mother and smiled. "Would you mind stepping out? I have to check a few things." My mother quickly nodded and left the room. When the door closed, Dr. Simon sat down next to me and asked with sharpened eyes, "Now that your mom's gone, why don't you tell me what's really going on? Your IBS is gone, and you've gained more weight than is normal. I've been doing this for a while, you know."

I was a bit startled at the intensity of Dr. Simon's voice, but what really caught me off guard was the question itself. I certainly didn't want to tell the only doctor I trusted that I was taking anabolic steroids, but I figured that Dr. Simon would figure it out—if he hadn't already. I told him everything, from how I had thought up the idea to use anabolic steroids to treat my IBS to how my skin hadn't blistered for nearly three months without the need for Dapsone. He listened carefully. To my own surprise, I also mentioned that since starting the steroids, I was feeling more stable. Never before had I mentioned stability to anyone or been able to gauge myself.

Dr. Simon met my eyes with a hard stare. I could tell that he wasn't happy I had tried something so dangerous without first consulting him, but there was a hint of curiosity. When he spoke, his voice was cold and his words chosen carefully. "You have put me in a horrible position, Kirk. I can't support your use of anabolic steroids. And at the dosage you are taking—are you even aware of the side effects?" He sighed as he shook his head. "I certainly can't write you a prescription."

"I know you can't," I interrupted him, sensing that he was growing more upset the longer he thought about what I had done. "And I would never ask you to, but the truth is that I've never felt better. As for the drugs, I can get them myself and won't ever ask you for a prescription. My source is good, and the only reason I didn't tell you, or anyone for that matter, was because I knew no one would approve, but the results …"

This time, Dr. Simon cut me off. Although he looked angry, I could see a glimmer of curiosity in his eyes. "So you haven't told anyone?" When I nodded, he continued. "I should drop you as a patient, but it's my job to help. Although I can't support what you're doing, I can't stop you. Since I can't control you, I have a responsibility to make sure you are safe." Dr. Simon leaned back in his chair, his hands resting on his small belly. "Are you willing to do biweekly blood tests and keep track of your IBS, Linear IGA, and mood swings?"

"Yes," I said quickly, sensing that although he didn't agree with what I was doing, he wasn't about to let me kill myself on his watch.

"If you slip up or do anything without consulting me …"

"I won't. You have my word."

Dr. Simon nodded, adding, "Then I'll try my best to keep you safe." Turning away from me, he opened the door and asked Suzie to get my mother. We sat quietly for a moment as we waited. I knew that Dr. Simon couldn't tell anyone what we had just discussed, so I was a bit curious as to why he had wanted to see my mother. When she entered, he wasted no time as he asked, "So, Jeanne, how have Kirk's mood swings been? And be honest." He was checking my story, which I just thought was intelligent.

My mother looked at me, wondering if she truly could be honest. I nodded, and my mother actually smiled. "He's been far more stable over the past four months, and he's even been able to work."

I could tell that Dr. Simon was both skeptical and worried, but he had Suzie write me up for a host of blood tests, put a smile on for my mother, and gave her a quick hug. "I want to see Kirk more regularly, so have Bonnie set up an appointment for next week." After my mother said that she would, Dr. Simon turned to me. "I'll see you soon." The look he gave me felt like a reminder that I had agreed to his demands and was not to cross him. I simply nodded as he turned and left the room.

After setting up my next appointment, my mother and I left. Looking down at the blood order, I was astonished at how many tests Dr. Simon had ordered. He wasn't kidding about making sure I was okay, and I didn't mind. He was the first person who knew about what I was doing, and over the next few years, he kept a very close eye on me. Strangely enough, our secret would eventually bring us closer together.

A full year had passed since I had started taking steroids, and I was aware that long-term use of anabolic steroids could cause problems. Eventually they did, but the problems were different from what I had expected. At first, the visits with Dr. Simon included a lecture that I should try and back off the steroids, but over time, as my IBS, skin problems, and bipolar continued to either remain in remission or improve, I could tell that Dr. Simon was growing more curious. As any good doctor would, he remained cautious and kept me busy with blood tests and mood charts.

As time went on, I began to become more aware of my moods. I still couldn't control them, but just being aware of what was going on was an entirely new experience. Also, my manic and depressive episodes did not come as often. Feeling better and continuing my research, trying to find any reason why anabolic steroids might actually help someone with bipolar, I decided it was time to take my experiment a step further. Like many bipolar patients, I had stopped taking my medications before, but this time I called Dr. Simon to get permission.

After a long talk, he decided that my lithium level, being slightly in the toxic range, could be lowered a very small amount. Following Dr. Simon's directions, I cut one of my four lithium pills into eight pieces, taking all but the single eighth. Essentially, Dr. Simon was lowering my total dosage by around three percent. He wouldn't let me lower my other drugs, as he wanted to see how I did with one at a time. While I was breaking apart one of my lithium pills, I didn't realize that my mother was standing behind me.

"What are you doing?" she asked, startling me as I quickly spun around to face her. "You know that you can't stop taking your medications."

I backed away from the table, showing my mom how many pieces I had divided the large pill into. "I'm not going to stop taking my medications, but I'm doing better, so I want to try and cut it down. I'm only lowering it by around three or four percent with Dr. Simon's permission." My mother's eyes began to tear up. I'm sure she was imagining me falling apart again.

"How about I make a deal with you?" I said to distract her from her thoughts. My mother looked back and forth from the cut-up pill to me, not saying anything. "Don't tell anyone that I'm cutting back my lithium, and if you or anyone else feels like I'm getting worse, I'll go back to 1,800 milligrams."

"Give me your word," my mother said, knowing that if I gave my word, I would never break it. I took pride in my sense of honor and had never broken my word to my knowledge. My mother knew this and was intelligent to ask.

"I give you my word. If I get worse, I'll up the dose." My mother walked over and hugged me, gripping me tightly. She didn't want me to get worse, but I could tell she wanted to believe I could get better. Later on, I learned that she thought if she had fought me I might have decided to stop all medication. In her way, she was trying to keep me safe. I didn't know until years later how much my decision had terrified and burdened her. I should never have asked her to keep such a large secret or given her the responsibility to try and watch me objectively. Surprising us both, however, I only continued to get better and more stable.

Although I was feeling better and more stable, I had yet to fully recover. My quality of life had increased immensely, and the heavy fog that made my mind feel slow and dull from the medications thinned a bit each time Dr. Simon allowed me to drop my dosage by a tiny increment. I kept up with my charts and blood tests, and at least once a week I asked my mother how she thought I was doing. As the rest of my family members believed that all the therapy and medications were finally working, my mother was trying her best to stay objective as I continued to lower my medications bit by bit.

On the weeks when I had been even a bit off, my mother would be very blunt, and we wouldn't lower my dosage. To her surprise, I didn't fight her. As the months passed and I continued to feel better, things were looking up. I felt smarter and less drugged, and I was even beginning to become more aware of my swings. My ability to sense my moods, however, did not give me any true control over them. During the months when I was lowering my medications, my swings didn't vanish. I did have a few brushes with mania and depression, but each swing was less severe and lasted a shorter time. My mother never panicked even though I know she was always waiting for me to fall beyond control. Fortunately, I never did.

I don't remember exactly how long I had been taking the anabolic steroids, but I had cut both my lithium and Lamictal down by nearly twelve percent and was doing very well mentally. I didn't know at the time, but my mother had talked to Dr. Simon, keeping him updated on how I was doing. I was in a particularly strange situation because my mother didn't know that I was experimenting with anabolic steroids while lowering my medications, but knowing that Dr. Simon was carefully watching me made my mother feel better.

Since I was remaining more stable as time went on, I felt I had to come clean with my mother, telling her what I had been taking. Her eyes widened with shock as she heard me explain that I, her only son, had been experimenting on myself. Her shock turned to anger as she felt like I hadn't told her the entire truth. I was honest, telling her that I had kept her in the dark so that she could judge my moods without thinking about another variable.

"I'm calling Dr. Simon," she said, picking up the phone with anger in her eyes.

"He already knows," I said, making her anger turn to surprise as she put down the phone. "I would've told you, but I wanted you to judge me without thinking about all the stories you hear in the media about steroids. I needed you to be completely objective."

I had glimpsed the pain I had caused Nicoal more than a year ago. This time, when I glimpsed the stress I had caused my mother, the clarity of my realization didn't fade. It was the first time I had seen how my actions affected others without the realization fading away. Walking over to my mother, I reached out and gave her a hug as she began to cry. Her tears were not caused from sadness as she squeezed me with her thin but strong arms. They were caused by joy. "Do you know how long it's been since you've given me a hug?" my mother asked. I didn't know the answer.

It is hard to look back and realize that whenever I was depressed or manic, I withheld affection. All my life, I had been so wrapped up with my own needs, seeing everyone in terms of what value they could add to my life, that I had never thought about their needs. When I wanted to get my way, I could read people, manipulating emotions and situations to gain what I wanted. The realization that I had not even given my own mother the love she deserved still deeply haunts me.

"I'll get better," was all I could think of to say. "I need you to keep what I just told you to yourself, as Chandi and Dad need to see me without knowing. I will tell them when it is time, but I need them to judge me just by my moods."

"I understand," my mother answered, her voice serious. She knew what I was trying to do.

I was glad that my mother knew, as it had been hard to keep my actions a secret from everyone but Dr. Simon. Dr. Simon was monitoring my health, my IBS and Linear IGA were both gone, and my broken mind was slowly beginning to heal. What I wasn't expecting was that I was one of the rare people whose blood wasn't designed for anabolic steroid use. The next few months nearly cost me my life.

When the symptoms first began, I hardly noticed them. I would feel hot and itchy over my entire body, but there was no rash or blisters. The feeling would fade as soon as I lifted weights or had to go out into the cold. Things slowly grew worse, and I often felt an incredible urge to scratch my back, chest, arms, and legs. I told my father of my symptoms, and he checked for a rash, but there was nothing to explain my symptoms. Usually, an intense itch was accompanied by some form of rash, so my symptoms were a bit mysterious.

Wondering if I was allergic to something, we checked the house. We looked at everything that might cause skin irritation. When the itch intensified, making me feel as if my skin were being pricked by thousands of red-hot needles, I knew something was wrong. Not wanting to bother Dr. Simon or feeling like it was serious, I tried researching my symptoms myself, but to no avail. When the burning no longer faded away and I began coughing, unable to stop, I knew I needed help. For the first time in my life, I called the doctor and made my own appointment.

My cough and symptoms worried my family. I would cough throughout the night. Sometimes my coughing would become so violent that the whites of my eyes would turn bright red, which looked terrifying and wasn't something I wanted my family to see. After two sleepless nights and two days of nonstop coughing, it was time for my doctor's appointment. I was planning on going alone, but my mother thought she should come in case Dr. Simon had any questions about my stability or medications. I actually think my willingness to go by myself shocked her. I still hadn't realized that I was acting like an adult.

This time, when Dr. Simon entered the room, he looked worried. I wasn't aware, but my face was red and my cough was high-pitched. It was obvious that I wasn't suffering from a normal cold. The first thing I noticed when Dr. Simon came into the room was that he was holding a large glass jug in one hand and a long tube with needles on both ends.

Moving past his nurse, Dr. Simon sat down at my side, lifting his stethoscope under my shirt as he listened to my lungs. In the years that I had been coming to see Dr. Simon, I had never seen him move so quickly. "Hold up your hand," he said, attaching a small clip over my right forefinger. While waiting for the machine to analyze my oxygen statistics, Dr. Simon put a blood pressure cuff over my left arm. When the small device on my finger beeped, showing that my blood was low in oxygen, Dr. Simon looked to Suzie. "His hematocrit is at a dangerous level. I need to draw his blood, so keep the cuff tight."

Suzie did as Dr. Simon asked as he rubbed my main vein with an alcohol swab. "So what is going on?" I asked.

"Your red blood cell count is so high that I am worried. We need to draw your blood to thin it. Just lie back," Dr. Simon answered before quickly sliding the thick needle into my arm. It stung, but I was used to needles. As the tube filled with my blood, Dr. Simon pushed the other side into the special glass jar, talking as my blood slowly drained out of my body. My blood was so thick and rich with red blood cells that it dripped into the jar instead of flowing. Dr. Simon was not pleased.

"I've been monitoring your blood levels for months now, but last week your tests concerned me, so I had the lab run a few more tests. Long story short, your erythropoietin is over ten times the normal level, and the mass and number of your red blood cells is far too high."

The relief I felt as my blood left my body was immense. My skin stopped burning, my cough vanished, and I felt as if a wave of energy were flowing into me. "I know what EPO is," I said. It was a topic I had quickly researched when studying the anabolic steroids. "I thought a high EPO count was a good thing."

"Some athletes use blood doping or anabolic steroids to increase their erythropoietin levels, but most people test around four to eleven. Your test came back at sixty-five. Although higher erythropoietin levels should enhance your endurance, a number that high puts you at risk of stroke, heart attack, and other issues. What you have is rare and not something I was expecting to see. We're just lucky that we caught it when we did." With my mother in the room, Dr. Simon was careful not to hint or give away that I was taking steroids.

"So you're saying that the anabolic steroids caused this?" I asked, seeing Dr. Simon's surprise that I had obviously told my mother. Just to make sure he felt comfortable talking, I added, "I told her everything, so feel free to talk."

"At first I thought that was the case, but your numbers are so high that I believe you had a preexisting issue. Although it is extremely rare, I went through your medical history and found that your red blood cell count has always been near a dangerous level. That is why I had your EPO tested as well as your red blood cells' mass. I was hoping I was wrong, but I believe you have always had what is called secondary polycythemia, or erythrocytosis. It can cause all your symptoms, and due to the altitude and how active you are, I believe the anabolic steroids exacerbated your condition. This means we have a major problem."

"So, I'm going to have to stop taking the anabolic steroids," I assumed, trying to remain calm at the news that the one thing that had helped temper my mood swings might not be an option any longer.

"Well, we have two major problems. First of all, from all your mother has told me, it seems that somehow, your bipolar has continued to fade away and your IBS and IGA are no longer problems. All this coincides with when you began taking the steroids. I don't pretend to know why, and frankly I still have a hard time believing it, but from everything I've seen and heard, you're doing better than ever, so I'd prefer not to have you stop. However—" Dr. Simon paused as he checked to see how full the jar was. "If you don't stop using them, your condition will either remain the same, get worse, or kill you. To be blunt, you're lucky you haven't already had a stroke or heart attack with your blood levels where they are."

"I can't stop using them," I said, not willing to give up on the one thing that had improved my life. My skin cleared up, I no longer needed Dapsone to keep my skin from blistering, I was free of my IBS, and my bipolar was continuing to improve. All the good I had experienced had occurred *after* I had started using anabolic steroids. To me, it seemed like too strong a coincidence to cast aside.

My mother had remained quiet since we got there, but she finally spoke up. "Dr. Simon, Kirk really is getting better. If the steroids have helped, as odd as that might be, is there anything we can do to avoid having Kirk stop? What about lowering the dose or taking his blood more often?"

Dr. Simon checked the bottle, making sure my blood was still flowing. "I can keep drawing his blood when his numbers get too high, but there are serious risks to that approach. To be honest, I'm not sure I want Kirk to stop taking the steroids, but I fear the risks of keeping him on them."

Suddenly I remembered a study I had recently come across. I nearly sat up with excitement as it could be a potential solution. "I read a study where a doctor was using a drug called Arimidex to raise men's testosterone instead of using anabolic steroids. Since I might not be able to keep taking testosterone, do you think that might be something worth trying?"

"Arimidex is an antiestrogen," Dr. Simon said, his mind clearly analyzing the idea as he pumped up the cuff around my arm to tighten it just a bit. "The idea is interesting. However, Arimidex would not raise your testosterone in comparison, nor do we know why the anabolic steroids are helping. When you first told me what you were doing, I would have bet my life that the steroids would've caused you to rocket into mania. To my surprise, you have grown more stable, which makes no sense to me. The third problem is that I can't write you a prescription for Arimidex."

When the glass jar was full, Dr. Simon removed the needle from my arm and bandaged the hole. I sat up, feeling better than I could express. "I promised you that I would never ask you to write a prescription. If I can get the Arimidex, do you think it's worth trying?"

Dr. Simon laughed and then caught himself before looking at my mother. "Your son is trying to give me a heart attack, isn't he?" Dr. Simon's joke had lightened the mood of the room as he looked at me. "Your cough is gone, and you look much better. As for your idea, I can't stop you from doing anything, but at this point, I feel it would be risky to try anything new. I am against the use of anabolic steroids, but for you—" Dr. Simon paused, not sure what to say. "I have no idea why they haven't made your bipolar worse, let alone better. I will monitor you and keep you safe, whatever decision you make, under one condition. I don't want you doing anything on your own without consulting me, and I want you to see another psychiatrist to monitor your bipolar. There is a chance that all this is simply a fluke, and I will not let anything happen to you on my watch."

With that, Dr. Simon left the room. I stared at the ceiling. For the first time in my life, my bipolar was growing easier to deal with. Had I not taken the risk with the nandrolone decanoate for my IBS, I wouldn't be feeling better. I didn't want my life to fall apart again, and I needed more research to support any change.

As I began to walk out of the room, my mother stopped me. "What are you going to do?"

"I've come this far, and I'm not going back to the way I was. I know I still have swings, but I think trying the Arimidex is the best option. I'll do some research and let Dr. Simon make the call. If it doesn't work, I can always go back on the anabolic steroids."

IV. RESEARCH, TRIAL, AND LUCK

I became frustrated after spending a few days looking for the study that had shown Arimidex to be a possible alternative for men seeking testosterone replacement therapy. It was gone. I did find some information that talked about it, but the original study had been removed. Although I couldn't find the study, I remembered the article well, and the theory was sound. I also did not feel that I had much of an option. Since the anabolic steroids, even at a lower dose, held greater health risks for me than for other individuals, I knew that I had to give Arimidex a try. The same source that had provided the anabolic steroids also had Arimidex. Knowing that I would get the real medication even though it was quite expensive, I took the plunge. I was finally feeling better, so I wasn't going to take more risks than needed.

Since the study I was interested in had been removed, I switched my research to the drug itself. As one of the more potent antiestrogens on the market, it was a popular choice with athletes who were coming down off of a steroid cycle. Bodybuilders and athletes used Arimidex to counteract a heavy steroid cycle, ensuring that there were no spikes in estrogen in an attempt to quickly boost their natural testosterone. Although there were some serious side effects for women, the drug had been designed for treating breast cancer when tamoxifen citrate was no longer effective. For men, there were also side effects, but most of the serious side effects were nothing compared to the bipolar medications that were already causing physical damage.

The medical community itself kept itself safely away from anything to do with anabolic steroids due to all the controversy surrounding steroids and sports. In many ways, this fact made me angry. I believed, especially after my own experience, that the endocrine system had great potential for treating bipolar and perhaps other mental disorders. That fact plus the fact that it had cleared up my IBS, my Linear IGA, and lupus and AIDS in other patients made me frustrated that more research was not being done.

In the end, I knew that I had to give the Arimidex a chance. If it didn't work, I would go back to the anabolic steroids. I felt that my life was worth risking to stave off the chaos that bipolar brought to every facet of my life. After getting Dr. Simon's permission and also telling my mother what we had decided, I took my first dose, swallowing a one-milligram tablet of Arimidex.

Although I had stopped taking the steroids, I still had to have my blood drawn every few weeks, missing only weeks when my iron was low. Dr. Simon had also prescribed oxygen for me to use when and if I felt it necessary. The only other option was to move away from Colorado and down to a lower altitude, but I couldn't uproot Nicoal as she was going to school. At Dr. Simon's request, I did not change any of my bipolar medications as everyone was worried about what might happen.

After I had been off of the steroids for three weeks, my IBS returned; however, it was less severe and painful than before and was very manageable. My skin had also remained smooth, with no sign that the blisters would return. I don't know how, but it appeared that the anabolic steroids had helped both my body and mind. What's more, when it came to mental stability, the Arimidex was much better.

Over the next few months I continued to have my blood taken when my red blood cell count rose too high and used oxygen daily. Although these were not good things to have to deal with, I would have gone through anything to experience the calm that was overtaking my mind. Not only did my mood swings come less frequently but also their intensity lessened noticeably. Slowly, my shattered mind, broken from years of delusions, depression, and explosive manic episodes, was beginning to heal. The better I became, the more obvious it was to everyone that something was working. My psychiatrists and Dr. Simon were startled with my progress and had no explanations as to why the Arimidex was working.

After a long while of watching me become more stable, Dr. Simon finally told me it was time to continue lowering my bipolar medications. Even with as much research as I had done, I still didn't know why the anabolic steroids had helped my bipolar, and even though I had made an educated choice to try Arimidex, Dr. Simon and I were both stumped as to why it was working. Bipolar was still thought to be incurable, yet mine was simply fading away.

After six months of titrating my bipolar medications, I found myself off all of them, although I continued to take clonazepam to treat my generalized anxiety, which remained. The fog that the medications had cast over my mind and all the side effects I had lived with for far too long were suddenly gone. My mood swings continued to fade away, and I began seeing through normal eyes for the first time. The colors were brighter, but more importantly I enjoyed them. Since childhood, I had always said my favorite color was black, but as the world no longer felt dark and twisted, I found a sense of awe when looking at bright and vibrant colors. For the first time in my life, free of bipolar, I understood what true happiness felt like, and I was moved.

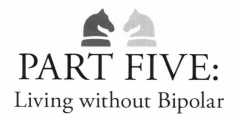

PART FIVE:
Living without Bipolar

:: Learning How to Live and Love a Normal Life ::

I. STRUGGLING TO COPE WITH NORMALITY

After I discontinued the use of anabolic steroids and switched to the antiestrogen Arimidex, my mind, which had once been broken and corrupted by bipolar, continued to heal rapidly. I still remembered Dr. Smith telling me that I might not ever lead a normal life, even with the use of bipolar medications. I agreed with him in part, for despite the dozens of mood-stabilizing and antipsychotic drugs I had tried, I hadn't been a functioning human being until after adding Arimidex to the mix.

After six months of taking the Arimidex, I was still showing no symptoms of mania or depression. I had slowly weaned off all my bipolar medications. The only medication that I was using to stabilize my moods was Arimidex, and it was amazing. Dr. Simon kept a close eye on me, still refusing to believe that my bipolar was in control. He wanted to believe, but the doctor inside him just couldn't accept what he was seeing. I didn't mind, for I was leading a normal life without bipolar swings.

What surprised me, however, was that the longer I remained stable the more aware of myself I became. As wonderful as it was to see the world and myself clearly, it was also painful, for I was suddenly aware of what most people would consider normal emotions. Throughout my life, bipolar had kept me from seeing anything but extremes, so I was not prepared. The better I became at analyzing myself, the more I realized who and what I used to be. To be candid, I wasn't prepared to face my past, nor was I prepared for a normal life. Whether or not I was ready, the challenge was coming at me head-on.

All my life, I had never faced things like fear, hope, or joy without bipolar twisting the emotions into an extreme. For example, I had never felt fear, just assumed I would die, and joy was always experienced as extreme bliss. This was true of all my emotions. These extremes had not only ruined relationships and robbed me of great opportunities but also shielded me from growing up. The sharper and more stable my mind became, the less I liked who I used to be and the harder it was to deal with being normal. Seeing the world like others did was not always easy, but I was willing to face any challenge to experience the stability and control I now felt. For the first time, although I was facing new challenges, I felt like I could determine my own destiny.

Although I was doing well, Dr. Simon, my psychiatrists, and my family continued to watch me carefully, worried that my recovery had been a fluke. In the absence of a shred of scientific data or a single study to support using an antiestrogen as a mood-stabilizer, everyone expected me to crash. I wasn't worried, however, as I was living for the first time without bipolar distorting my vision. No one could've known it was working better than I, and what I saw and felt on a daily basis only confirmed that I was getting better. I couldn't explain what I was experiencing, for it was a new experience for me, and I was the only one living it.

Because everyone expected me to crash, everyone was extra sensitive. When I experienced a hard day that made me feel a bit grumpy or a great day that raised my spirits, everyone would ask if I had taken my medication and was okay. I disliked the question, and it took me time to realize that the only reason my family members asked was because they cared. What startled me was that until then, I had not really understood how much I was loved. Even my perception of love had been distorted by bipolar.

Even as I struggled to understand all the changes I was going through as I got better, I never thought that my family would have a hard time adjusting to the new me. Now free of my wild swings, I was focused and calm. It was strange to discover that I was not the comedian I thought I was but was actually a very serious and passionate person. My manic episodes had always deluded me into believing that I was a carefree joker, but the truth was that it was the bipolar swings that made me carefree. It was strange to realize that I didn't even know who I really was, but discovering myself was interesting.

My recovery affected everyone around me. My mother was so used to taking care of me when I wasn't able to take care of myself that she kept preparing food for me without knowing that I had already made myself lunch. It wasn't only my mother who was having a hard time adjusting to the absence of my bipolar; everyone I was close with had formed some way to survive dealing with my irrational explosions and deep depressions. My sister, used to trying to lift my spirits when I was down, continued to spend her hard-earned money buying me gifts. My father found it strange when I joined everyone at the dinner table and talked instead of vanishing into the basement. The first time I asked my father how his day had been, his eyes widened with shock, making me realize that I had never taken an interest in anyone's life but my own.

Nicoal had a very hard time adjusting to my stability. Although she was used to seeing both my mania and depression, she focused on our best moments, which always took place when I was first becoming manic. Like everyone who was close to me, Nicoal had blocked out many of our worst times and clung to the memories of when I couldn't stop laughing, joking, or telling funny stories. With no more mania, I didn't laugh or joke the way I used to, leading her to constantly doubt my happiness. No longer imbalanced and truly happy for the first time in my life, I realized that no matter how many times I tried to explain that I was happy, it would take time for everyone to adjust to the new me. The hardest part for me was being reminded of who I used to be and facing the fact that my instability had forced the people I loved to change their lives in an attempt to survive living with me.

One thing was very clear about my situation: there was no one to help guide me. I read countless memoirs and books about bipolar, but I couldn't find anyone who was in the same situation. Even though I knew my wife, family, and friends loved me, I felt very alone at times and knew that I would have to adapt to a "normal" life on my own. After tasting what real stability was like, I didn't think I could survive if my bipolar returned.

The only problem was that the Arimidex was expensive. Since I was getting hospital-grade medication from the black market, the medication was actually more expensive than if I had purchased it from a pharmacy. Not only was I faced with the challenge of understanding my new life but also my recovery was being threatened for the first time as I realized I just couldn't afford to continue taking the medication.

Desperate to find a solution before going back on the anabolic steroids, I began researching other antiestrogens. When I contacted my source to see if there was any way I could get the Arimidex at a lower cost, my source suggested that I take a look at a drug called tamoxifen citrate. With tamoxifen citrate also being an antiestrogen at a fraction of the price, I used all my spare time to research the drug. Although tamoxifen citrate was also used in the treatment of breast cancer, it had a different way of lowering the estrogen in my body. What surprised me was reading the comments left by bodybuilders who had tried taking a break from their steroids without using tamoxifen citrate or Arimidex. Many of them reported feeling depressed, crying and even contemplating suicide. Men who had used the tamoxifen citrate, however, did not suffer from depression and reported feeling very stable even after a heavy cycle. Since my mind was finally beginning to heal, I didn't want to take any risks, but I was quickly running out of money and needed to make a decision before I ran out of my Arimidex.

I scheduled an appointment to see Dr. Simon; I wasn't about to make any decisions before consulting him. Although I had caused my body considerable harm with my self-experimentation, Dr. Simon had slowly begun to trust my research and respect my mind and ideas. Even after watching my bipolar vanish, he fully admitted that the medical professional inside him was not ready to accept that Arimidex had stabilized my moods. In fact, out of everyone in my life, he was perhaps most concerned that my bipolar would come back.

After signing in, filling out paperwork, and being brought back to one of the exam rooms, I sat down on the examination table and suddenly realized that it was the first time I had come to the doctor by myself. It was certainly the first time I had ever filled out any paperwork. To most people, this would not be a big deal, but I realized that I was becoming self-sufficient.

Dr. Simon walked into the room and sat down. "I just talked with your psychiatrist and your family. Everyone says that you feel and act like a completely different person, but the truth is that I'm worried. You realize that we aren't out of the woods yet, don't you?" I nodded, knowing that no doctor would believe I was in the clear until a few years had passed. "So, have you had any dark thoughts or felt even a bit manic?"

"No. I've actually been doing really well," I answered truthfully. "I've been saving as much money as I can. I haven't missed a day of work, and as for my moods …" I paused for a second, realizing that I truly was aware of my moods. I didn't have to think about whether I had felt any depression or mania. I knew that I hadn't. "The bipolar is gone."

"I have been practicing medicine since your mother was a child, and I can honestly say that you are the first true mystery that has walked into my office." Dr. Simon wasn't smiling as he added, "And I'm not fond of mysteries."

Getting to business, Dr. Simon ran his hand through his thin gray hair as he asked, "So, what did you want to talk to me about?"

"I've been researching another antiestrogen."

Dr. Simon cut me off before I could finish. "The Arimidex appears to be working. Why are you still researching?"

"I'd prefer not to stop taking the Arimidex, but I just can't afford the medication." As Dr. Simon sighed, understanding where I was coming from, I continued. "The drug I've been researching is much cheaper than Arimidex, and it's actually been used in official trials to treat mania. There are no studies that show it works as a mood stabilizer, but I've read enough to believe it might work just as well as the Arimidex."

"And what were the results of the trials?"

"They were not conclusive but not completely negative." I explained what I had found, stated my case, and waited for Dr. Simon to respond.

Dr. Simon gave another small sigh. "Tamoxifen is another antiestrogen used to treat breast cancer, and I still don't have a clue as to why Arimidex has helped you. Do you really want to risk your stability by changing anything?"

I was about to answer when an odd sensation washed over me. As my mind grew sharper and my life finally got back on track, there were moments where I was overcome by emotions that I didn't understand and had never felt before. I knew in theory what anger, joy, fear, and sadness were, but the truth was that I had never truly experienced any real emotions until recently. Understanding and handling new and unfamiliar emotions was the most trying and difficult challenge that I faced in learning to lead a normal life.

Dr. Simon just sat there, waiting for me to answer as I tried to figure out what I was feeling. All my life, decisions had been easy. I had lived without any fear or regret to hold me back from making rash choices, so when I wasn't able to immediately answer, I felt confused. What I was really feeling, however, was doubt and fear. I didn't know it at the time, but I did know that I didn't like how I felt. Taking a breath, I finally answered. "I don't want to risk anything, but money is tight, and I don't have a choice. I can get tamoxifen from the same person who is supplying the Arimidex. Honestly, I don't know …"

I paused again, frustrated that I was having a hard time deciding on what was best. I had done my research and felt like tamoxifen citrate was the right choice, yet I kept wondering what might happen if I was wrong. I had never hesitated before, so the feeling was a bit strange. Overwhelmed with emotions that I was not equipped to deal with, I wondered if something was wrong.

Dr. Simon was watching me closely, analyzing my hesitation, which I had never displayed before. "Do you think it is the smart choice? I have been against every move you have made, but you have done well. If you're feeling doubt, just know that I'll support whatever decision you make and monitor you. If the tamoxifen doesn't work as well, you call me at the first sign of trouble. Don't wait. Do you understand?"

"I do," I said, realizing that Dr. Simon had seen my emotions before I had. I had never felt doubt before, and I didn't like it. I had never cared what others thought, so I was surprised at how much Dr. Simon's words meant. My ego had always had two settings, making me believe that I was either godlike or worthless. Dr. Simon's statement had made me feel more confident, and I liked that feeling much better than doubt. "I'll get the tamoxifen and call you before I change anything."

Dr. Simon nodded. "I want you to give me a call whenever you need to. Do you have my cell phone number?"

I knew that Dr. Simon kept his cell phone number secret, as all doctors needed and deserved some personal time and privacy, so I felt honored when he told me his number, watching as I entered the number into my phone. After I had entered his number, he handed me his cell. "I'm horrible with these things. Just put your number in and call me if anything changes."

"I will," I said with a slight smile as I quickly entered my information into his phone. Somehow, even though I had caused Dr. Simon more worry than he deserved, I had earned his respect. I knew he was still waiting for things to go south, but that wasn't going to happen. I may have felt doubt about trying something other than Arimidex, but I knew my mind was healing. If it was indeed the antiestrogen that had freed me from bipolar, then I had to believe that the tamoxifen would also work. This was flawed logic as the two medications had very different modes of action, but they were at least considered related drugs.

After saying good-bye to Bonnie, Suzie, and Dr. Simon, I left the office and walked to my car. The air was fresh, and the cool breeze lightly stung my cheeks. Even though Dr. Simon had given me the green light for switching from the Arimidex to the tamoxifen citrate, I couldn't shake the vision of who I used to be. For the first time in my life, I felt doubt and fear, making me wonder if there was a way I could make more money to stay on the Arimidex. In the past I had made life-changing decisions without a second thought, but now that I was balanced, I was struggling to trust my own research.

Getting into the car, I put my seat belt on before raising my hands to my face. I had never realized the extent to which bipolar had shielded me from feeling emotions. The emotions I had felt when manic or depressed had always been twisted, extreme, and fleeting, but the doubt I felt that day was like a splinter I couldn't pluck from my mind. Unable to shake the feeling, I began to understand that I was facing a difficult time of reflection.

Ever since I had started taking the Arimidex, my brain had grown sharper, more stable, and calmer, so feeling caught up in an emotion I didn't recognize was disconcerting. Because I was growing more aware of myself with each passing day, I had come to believe that I knew how to control my emotions. The truth, however, kept coming to the forefront: I had never experienced real or normal emotions before. I might have been free of bipolar, but I quickly realized that I had a long way to go before I could claim a full recovery.

Taking a deep breath, I started the car and turned the radio on. Although I couldn't shake the self-doubt I was feeling, I knew that I would eventually have to make a decision. When I returned home, I made a call to my contact and ordered a two-month supply of tamoxifen citrate. I wasn't sure if I would try it or not, but I figured the decision would be easier when the medication came.

A week later, the tamoxifen citrate arrived in the mail. My father walked into the kitchen, and saw me holding a bottle of Arimidex in one hand and tamoxifen citrate in the other. Intellectually I understood the definitions and effects of every human emotion, but I was finally beginning to feel them. At the moment, I was experiencing doubt again, but there was something new that made me feel jumpy. I didn't know what the emotion was, but it was disconcerting. Knowing theoretically about emotions and experiencing them were completely different things.

"You look like you're holding a bomb," my dad joked, his voice startling me. "What are you doing, and why are you so pale?"

I turned to look at my father, answering him truthfully. "I can't make up my mind." I sighed, frustrated that I couldn't make a decision. It was the first time I could remember struggling to commit. As my stability had continued, I had eventually told the entire family about what I was doing, so my dad was aware of the antiestrogens. "I don't get it, Dad. I did my research, but I keep wondering if I'm wrong."

My father walked over and looked at both medications before patting me on my shoulder. "Son, it's normal to doubt and worry, especially when your life is finally coming together."

Ever since talking with Dr. Simon about switching medications, I had been struggling to identify what I was feeling. Since I had never worried about myself, others, or my actions, my father's analysis of my emotions hit home. Looking away from the medications, I looked to my father. "How do I make such a big decision?"

Sensing that I was confused, my dad took both bottles of medication out of my hands and placed them on the kitchen counter. "Everyone deals with doubt and fear, son. You just can't let it control you. I can't tell you what to do, but I can tell you to trust your research and your gut. If the tamoxifen doesn't work as well, you can always switch back to the Arimidex. I'll help pay for it if I can." At the time, my parents were struggling, so his offer was beyond generous.

With no way to know if the tamoxifen citrate would be as effective as the Arimidex, I experienced my first moment in which bipolar would've made things easier. Realizing how emotionally stunted I was surprised me. Taking my father's advice, I trusted myself, repeating my father's words: "I can always switch back to the Arimidex." With that, I lifted the bottle of tamoxifen citrate from the counter, opened the bottle, and tipped it until a single tablet fell into my palm. "Thanks for the talk, Pops."

"Any time," he said with a gentle smile before walking away, leaving me alone in the kitchen.

It had never been clearer that adapting to normal life was going to be far more difficult than I had first thought. However, in many ways, as much as I hated feeling doubt or fear, I loved the truth of the emotions. I had lived a sheltered life for far too long, and I was ready to grow up and experience the world the way I was supposed to.

Switching to tamoxifen citrate had been a calculated risk that had worried everyone, but I had been taking the medication and remaining stable for two months. Everyone, including Dr. Simon, was growing increasingly confident that I had made the right choice. Although the two medications had very different methods of reducing the body's estrogen, they both worked. How they worked, however, was still a mystery that I wanted to solve.

II.   FACING AND EXPERIENCING REAL EMOTIONS

It is, and always will be, strange for me to look back and realize that all my life I had never experienced real emotions. I use the word "real" because I can't think of a better word. It wasn't that I hadn't felt anger, hatred, or bliss, for at the peaks of my mania or depression I had certainly acted out those emotions, but they had always been tainted and exaggerated by my twisted reality. As my mind grew sharper and I became more self-aware, I began to realize that I had never truly enjoyed watching a movie, opening presents, looking at the stars, or even having relationships. Even though I realized that every memory involving emotion was distorted, I still wasn't prepared for how my newly normal mind would experience and deal with emotions.

Some emotions, like joy, happiness, and love, were strong enough to make my eyes tear up. It was always easier to handle the positive emotions. They were indescribably vivid, affecting, true, and alluring. Every time I laughed, the world seemed brighter and warmer. In many ways I was like a child, overwhelmed and surprised with how powerfully a calm and free mind experienced emotions. Even though negative emotions like stress, fear, anger, and doubt were much harder to manage and control, mostly because they made me feel horrible, *feeling* real emotions, bad or good, was intoxicating. Since bipolar had only allowed me to taste the most extreme emotions, realizing how broad and varied real emotions were was very daunting and exciting.

For a time I was doing well, learning to let go of anger and enjoy the positive emotions, but when I was first hit with regret I was truly overwhelmed. Hatred and love seemed easy to understand compared to regret. Despite all the poor choices I had made in my life, bipolar had always kept me from looking back. Knowing there was no way to understand and accept my past without delving into it with an open mind, I was forced to look at the animal I used to be. It was more painful than I like to admit.

Now free of bipolar and able to look at my past and future with a startling clarity and understanding, I was very aware that I had never been in control. Yet knowing that I was not thinking with a normal mind during many of my most radical choices and actions did not lessen the guilt, pain, and horror I felt when looking at my past. When I was sober from my bipolar, my past was extremely painful to reflect upon. I had ruined countless friendships, demolished all but one romantic relationship, and passed up some amazing financial opportunities. Knowing that was hard to take. At least my swings kept me from realizing the impact of my actions. Eventually, I realized that I had one of two choices; I could let my past overwhelm me, letting my regret overrun my life, or I could let go of my past and appreciate the good and the bad that had led me to where I was: stable, successful, married, and happy.

Unlike with many of the new emotions I was experiencing, I couldn't sit back and let go of the regret I felt. I needed to take action, so I made a list of everyone whom I had wronged and began making calls. During my calls to more people than I like to admit, I never talked about bipolar, focusing only on apologizing for my actions. Some of the calls were extremely hard to make, but every time someone forgave me I felt a slight weight slide from my shoulders. I was looking for two things: forgiveness for my actions and the ability to start a new life that I was proud of. It took a long time, but eventually I began to accept my old life as part of who I was. Although I could never make up for what I had put my family and friends through, I was committed to trying. Finally learning how to let go of my regrets was a big step for me. The process helped me to understand who I used to be, who I wanted to be, and that I was lucky to be alive.

The better I got at recognizing, analyzing, and reacting calmly to the constant stream of new emotions, the more I appreciated being free of bipolar. Although bipolar protected me from many negative emotions and left me free to act without fear, doubt, or regret, feeling something real was so much more fulfilling. It had taken twenty-nine years to feel alive, but it was worth the wait. Normal life was so much sweeter with the knowledge of what it felt like to be ruled by rash thoughts and violent actions.

I was bipolar free, and although life wasn't always easy, I loved it. If I die early from the damage I caused to my body during my research, I would gladly trade my remaining life for the few years that I have recently been blessed to live.

III.   EVOLVING RELATIONSHIP DYNAMICS

Reflecting on my past, I felt ashamed of the person I used to be. This quickly led me to focusing on and centering my life around kindness and understanding. Although there were brief moments when I had been kind and thoughtful in my past, they were so rare that I felt the need to catch up. I had been living only for myself, so it wasn't a surprise that the list of people who had put up with me was extremely short.

During my life I had chased away so many great people, terrifying some and breaking the hearts of others. I wanted to make those who still stood by me proud. The first real problem I found about trying to be a good person was that I had established bad habits.

Due to the paranoia I experienced during my manic episodes, I had developed a sense that everyone was out for something or working against me. Since I was always looking out only for myself, it was no surprise that I had thought others worked the same way. Some of the habits that I had developed for self-preservation were hard to unlearn. Lying, for example, was second nature, and I had honed my ability to read and manipulate others before they could do the same to me. My dark view of the world had twisted me into a dark individual, but I now had a second chance.

After I had finally learned to manage my emotions with some level of understanding, it was frustrating when my old habits subconsciously lashed out. It felt as if every time I was getting the knack of being normal, a new twist or surprise would catch me off guard. I admit that no one can be perfect, but I was just trying to be better, and it was surprisingly hard. Even after more than a full year without a hint of bipolar showing through, I still caught myself manipulating my relationships. In the past, I had done so because I believed it was an act of survival. After I knew better, it was infuriating that lying and manipulating had become instinctual. I didn't want to lie anymore, for there was no need, and I wanted nothing more than to be a good person.

When I was a child, I remember that one of my best friends had a problem with cursing, so his mother made him put a penny in a jar every time he cursed. It had worked for my friend, so I figured that I would start a jar, adding a dollar whenever I caught myself manipulating, lying, or even gossiping. Needless to say, the jar filled up quickly as I struggled to change the person bipolar had molded me into. My determination, however, never wavered. Unlike in the past, when mania sent my brain into overdrive or depression held me back, I felt focused and in control. It was finally possible to change.

Very aware of the person I used to be and how bipolar had affected me, I did not like knowing that every action I had ever taken had been done with the sole intent of personal gain. I was slowly fixing the way I treated others, but it hit me that I was still doing it for myself. For so long, I had been so oblivious to other peoples' needs that I hadn't even thought about becoming a more giving individual. I certainly knew how to read others, so I decided to use that ability to help those I cared about. After spending my life feeding off of others, I thought it was my turn to give back.

The better I became at understanding my own motives and the needs of my friends, family, and wife, the better and more enjoyable each relationship became. Day by day I was growing more kind and gentle, slowly polishing the person I used to be into something I would be proud of. I was also working to be a better son, brother, friend, and husband. I admit that I made mistakes, but the more effort I put in the more all of my relationships, both personal and professional, strengthened.

That year was the first time I had acted in a selfless way without consciously thinking about it. My mother had made quite a feast for Thanksgiving, and for the first time I had enjoyed the holiday, eating with everyone and talking instead of hiding in my room, avoiding conversation. Seeing how happy everyone was made me realize that I had never truly enjoyed holidays or vacations. Worse, I realized that I had viewed them as obligations that I was forced into, typically ruining every occasion when our family did something together. Even Christmas, regardless of whether I was manic or depressed, always felt like a chore. Of course I looked forward to opening presents, but there were only so many presents. When I was done opening my gifts, I had always disappeared in my room, playing by myself. I rarely showed any appreciation for the gifts that I had been given. However, that year I was looking forward to Christmas, and not because I wanted something, but because I had gone shopping for everyone else for the first time in my life and was excited to give everyone their gifts.

I'm sad to admit that prior to that occasion, I can only think of three gifts that I had gone out and purchased for someone else. There was the engagement ring for my wife, a pearl necklace I had bought my sister when I was in high school, and a small stuffed animal for my mother. All the gifts that had supposedly come from me, my mother had picked out and wrapped for me every Christmas. Intent on making our family holiday special, I had even purchased wrapping paper. However, since I had never wrapped a present before, I didn't do the best job. Although my presents looked as if they had been wrapped by a two-year-old, I didn't care. It was also the first Christmas since I had been free of bipolar.

Three days after Thanksgiving, I waited patiently for everyone to go to bed. After making sure Nicoal was asleep, I carefully crawled out of bed, quietly grabbing my bag of poorly wrapped presents from my closet before walking upstairs. Setting the bag down, I tiptoed through the kitchen and quietly entered the garage.

Since I was a child, we had always kept our artificial Christmas tree in the garage. It was carefully and tightly wrapped in a large box that was long and wide, making it difficult to carry alone. I had watched my mother and father take out the tree every year, but couldn't remember ever helping without throwing a fit. This year would be different. Lifting the tree and hoisting it over my shoulder before carefully and quietly walking back inside, I nearly slipped on the kitchen floor but caught myself. It never even dawned on me that had I been helping every year, my mother and father wouldn't have needed to work so hard.

Opening the box as quietly as I could, I pulled out each piece of the tree, checking that the wires weren't tangled. Piece by piece, I assembled the tree, checking to make sure it wasn't off center. I wanted everything to be perfect and was determined to make it happen. The entire time I was putting the tree together, I had a silly grin on my face. For the first time, I was excited to decorate the tree and stack presents beneath it. I was even more excited to surprise my family and wife.

When I was finished, I stood there, finally understanding the magic of the holidays. It wasn't about presents or getting what I wanted, nor was it an obligation. The holidays were about appreciating everything I had and showing compassion and love to those I cared for. Cleaning up the box and putting it back into the garage, I had one thing left to do. Bringing my bag of presents over to the tree, I carefully placed the gifts I had personally wrapped under the tree.

Stepping back, I smiled, but the joy I felt quickly faded as I realized it was the first time I had done something wonderful without first having an agenda. As my mind swirled with memories of the past, the moment was bittersweet. I couldn't think of a single vacation or holiday that I had not ruined for my family. I wanted to believe that I was mistaken, but I knew I wasn't. The worst of the Christmas memories almost brought me to tears. I had been twelve, and before even opening my first present, I had lost my temper for a reason I couldn't remember. What stood out in my mind was that I had told my mother, father, and sister that I hated them before knocking over the tree and breaking my mother's favorite ornament.

Overwhelmed at the idea that I could have ever been so cruel, I sat down on the floor, my eyes locked on the tip of the tall Christmas tree, which was lit by the gentle moonlight shining in through our front windows. Overcome with guilt, I wondered if there would ever come a time when I could forgive myself for what I had done to those I cared most about.

"What are you doing up?" I heard my mother ask as she came out of her bedroom. Her voice quickly faded away as she looked down and saw me sitting in front of the tree. "You put up the tree."

I looked up and nodded, realizing that her voice had shaken as she spoke. She wasn't upset that I had awakened her; she was shocked at what she was looking at. "It was supposed to be a surprise, but since you're up, do you want to hang the first ornament?"

My mother stood at the top of the stairs for a long while, staring first at the tree and then back to me. After a long pause, she realized that I had asked her a question and nodded quickly before walking quietly down the stairs. Since it was late and I was hardly sleepy, I expected my mother to ask if I was feeling a bit manic, but she simply walked over to me and reached out her arms, repeating what she had already said. "You put up the tree."

"Yes," I responded as I gave my mother a big hug. "I just thought I would get it done so everyone else could just enjoy it."

My mother let go of me and walked over to the tree, noticing the presents I had set out around the base. When she turned back around, my mother's eyes were about to tear as she spoke. "You've never put up the tree before," she said as she pointed to the presents, adding, "And the presents."

When I saw my mother next to the tree with her eyes filled with tears, all I could think of was that I had broken the ornament that she had enjoyed since she was a child. Both of her parents had passed away when she was young, and that ornament was not replaceable. Needing to escape from the guilt I felt, I walked over to my mom, putting my hand on her shoulder as she stared at the tree with childlike awe. "I'm sorry that I broke your ornament."

My mother laughed as she turned to face me. She was crying, but her face was bright and filled with joy. "I don't care. This is worth a thousand ornaments."

I hadn't known how much my mother had wanted me to enjoy holidays and birthdays. As she took hold of me and cried tears of joy, I felt my past vanish, if only for that moment. At that moment, even though I was still struggling to understand who I was, I knew that it felt good to bring joy to others. It may have taken me twenty-nine years to give my family the Christmas they deserved, but I figured it was better late than never.

The next day, everyone was in good spirits, but the revelation that I had not a single memory in which I had not ruined an important occasion was still bitter. Refusing to let my past ruin the day, I put on a smile and swore that I would continue getting better. I had only been normal for a year. I felt like a child experiencing everything for the first time, but that wouldn't stop me from becoming a good man. Aware that I was a work in progress, I was finally beginning to understand who I wanted to be and how I wanted to be remembered.

IV.   A SECOND CHANCE AND A NEW PURPOSE

Long before I had begun taking Arimidex, my mother had talked me into going to a few bipolar support groups. I had been against the idea, thinking that I was too good to waste my time talking about my problems with a bunch of strangers. After a few weeks of refusing to try, I gave in. To my surprise, I ended up making quite a few friends. One of the people—I'll call him Tony—had so much in common with me that we became quite close. Tony, like me, was suffering from an extreme case of bipolar, and we shared many of the same passions and problems. Neither of us could hold down a job or keep ourselves from sabotaging our romantic relationships. Tony was four years older than I, and I now know that he was a reflection of my future.

Tony was missing his top teeth due to a bar fight. His stories and struggles were always familiar, but somehow I had avoided jail and many other unpleasant events while Tony hadn't. Like mine, Tony's manias would tear his world apart, but he was always caught and punished while I had somehow escaped unscathed from similar situations. For a time, Tony and I were very close, but when I began getting better, our commonalities began to vanish. After I had been taking Aridimex for six months, Tony and the others in the bipolar group asked me what medications I was taking, seeing how well I was doing and wanting to feel some form of control. I remembered the desperation they felt. No one wants to suffer from bipolar, and everyone in the group, especially the more severe cases like Tony and myself, were always searching for answers and the ability to live a normal life. As much as I wanted to tell everyone what I was taking and what I had discovered, I didn't want anyone to take the same risks that had almost killed me. I also had no idea whether my treatment program would work on others, although I believed in my research and thought there was true potential.

As time went on and the bipolar that had ruled my life continued to vanish, I was never more aware of the second chance I had been given than when I was talking with Tony. While my life and relationships continued to heal and improve, Tony's life was being eaten away due to his bipolar. Every time he lost another job due to his mania or he flew to another country believing he was too important to live in normal society, it was like I was looking into a mirror of my past. I do not like to use the words insane or crazy, but the more my mind healed the more I realized just how insane I used to be. Watching Tony made me wonder why I had been given a second chance when everyone else I knew who was bipolar was suffering. Bipolar had made me into a selfish, egotistical, and delusional monster, making me wonder why I was getting a second chance.

When Tony flew to California, believing he had figured out a new math that would change the world, I knew that I couldn't keep my discovery a secret. I didn't deserve a second chance to reinvent myself just so I could watch others like me continue to self-destruct. I knew that somehow I had to figure out if my discovery would work on others suffering from bipolar. With no credentials, however, I was just another bipolar individual. I would sound completely delusional if I tried to tell any professional that I had found a cure that science insisted did not exist.

Knowing that no one would listen to me, I called the only person

I thought could help. Dr. Simon agreed to meet with me. To this day, I still believe that Dr. Simon wanted to get to the bottom of my recovery as badly as I did. Although he had been skeptical at first, I was approaching him after eighteen months of stability, making my recovery more medically valid and all the more mysterious.

Later that week I drove to Dr. Simon's office and we sat down in private to talk. Dr. Simon had become a friend and a mentor, but more importantly, he was the only person who had seen my recovery. Dr. Simon had seen me more often than my psychiatrists and was the only one I had entrusted with every risk and experiment I had tried in a desperate attempt to heal my broken mind. As we both sat down, he straightened his tie and smiled. "You're looking good," he said, gesturing to my button-down shirt and slacks. "You realize that only a year ago I never saw you cleanly shaven or wearing anything but sweats?"

Dr. Simon brushed back his thinning silver hair and asked, "So, why did you want to meet?"

"Well, I'm not sure how to start," I began, deciding to simply dive in and ask. "I believe that the Arimidex or tamoxifen citrate will work on other people suffering from bipolar. However, I'm aware that because I have no credentials, no one will listen. So, to be blunt, I need help proving that I'm right. I want to help people escape bipolar so they can live a fulfilling life. The torture I felt and the reality I now enjoy … I just can't sit by without trying to help others."

Dr. Simon's smile flattened as he met my eyes with his own, thinking. "There is a possibility that the antiestrogens would work on others, but legally I can't do anything. I'd like to, but the liability is beyond what I can support."

Picking up the folder that was sitting at my side, I handed it to Dr. Simon and let him read before I explained. When I realized that I couldn't keep my recovery a secret, I had seen a lawyer, asking what possible options Dr. Simon might have. The lawyer had drawn up consent forms, explaining that Dr. Simon could use them to treat someone who had tried everything and had run out of options. Although his patients' experiences wouldn't be considered clinical data, if we could build up enough case studies showing that the medication worked, perhaps we would have a chance to get a clinical trial started. "I spoke to a lawyer before coming to meet you. If someone is suffering from bipolar and they are out of options, you can legally prescribe tamoxifen or Arimidex as long as they are fully informed of all potential risks and sign the informed consent form."

Dr. Simon looked over the papers and sighed before looking back to me. "Let me ask you something."

"Sure," I said as I nodded. "Shoot."

"I admit that you have surprised me, but I must ask, when you are finally stable and your professional and personal life are beginning to come together, why are you interested in trying your method of treating bipolar on anyone else?"

It was a fair question, and I was surprised by how easily my answer came. "Because now that I am better, I can't stand by and watch others suffer as I did. If there is even a chance that the antiestrogens could work on others, I couldn't live with myself if I didn't try. I am willing to help in any way I can, but I can't do it on my own."

Dr. Simon looked out the window and took a deep breath before returning his gaze to me. "I need to talk to my lawyer and get more detailed information, but I will see what I can do. You understand that I'm not promising anything, don't you?"

"I do," I said as I stood up. I was aware of the stress I had caused Dr. Simon when I had first begun to experiment, and I certainly wasn't going to push him now, especially after all he had done for me. "Thanks for everything," I added as I reached out and shook his hand.

A month later, Dr. Simon began to treat a few extreme cases of bipolar with tamoxifen citrate. He would have prescribed Arimidex, but because he was seeing the patients for free and providing the medication, he chose tamoxifen citrate because of its low cost. Together, Dr. Simon and I decided that we would approach treating others just as we had approached my own treatment. Each patient he wrote a prescription for had to be officially diagnosed with bipolar and working with a trained psychiatrist. As always, Dr. Simon wanted his patients to be safe.

Most importantly, all the subjects had to continue taking their bipolar medications, not cutting the doses unless they first talked to Dr. Simon, and were required to keep mood and medication charts. He also gave all the patients and their family members my phone number. Dr. Simon wanted me to coach them since I had been the first person to use an antiestrogen as a mood stabilizer. I was trained to not give any medical advice; if that was needed, the family or patient was to immediately contact Dr. Simon or a psychiatrist.

As patients slowly lowered their other medications and began to improve, they would call me with questions. Although everyone was told that I had no medical or counseling degree, family members and patients preferred to talk to me because they knew I understood what they were going through. More importantly, I could explain moods, triggers, and actions in a way that made sense. Now I knew why I had been given a second chance—to help everyone find the peace and joy I now lived with.

As time went on and the patients continued to improve, Dr. Simon and I both knew that there was some connection between the endocrine system and bipolar. Not only were many of the patients living stable lives without taking traditional bipolar medications, but they were also excelling at life. Their main problems were about dealing with normal emotions and stability. Like me, they struggled to understand their minds once their illness began receding. Luckily, I could help them understand what they were going through.

After spending countless hours talking to patients and family members, I was asked to write the story of how I overcame being bipolar. Dr. Simon and I were convinced the new method worked, and I decided that my story was worth writing. As much as I hope my book causes a stir in the medical world and a drive for new research, I feel blessed every day that I somehow escaped bipolar and am now helping others do the same. To everyone who has ever dealt, directly or indirectly, with this illness, I hope with all my heart that my story instills in you a sense of hope and courage.

There is a cure, and everyone should have a second chance.

Made in the USA
San Bernardino, CA
05 March 2013